ADVANCE PRAISE
FOR *COUNTERPUNCH*:

"The writing is very engaging, and ideal for the messages you are trying to convey. It's tough to make dry medical information entertaining, but you are succeeding admirably."

Dr. David Riley,
Co-founder, InMotion, Cleveland, OH

●

"Gil and Struby are dear friends and compatriots in the fight against PD. They have devoted themselves to making life better for their fellow PwPs and care partners. *Counterpunch* provides inspirational and unflinchingly honest insight into their lives. Definitely a worthwhile read for anyone who aspires to understand the reality of living with PD."

Kirk Hall,
Denver PD advocate and author of "Carson and His Shaky Paws Grampa," "Carina and Her Care Partner Gramma" and with Benzi Kluger, "Window of Opportunity: Living with the Reality of Parkinson's and the Threat of Dementia."

●

"*Counterpunch* is terrific—comprehensively informative, personally open, and invitational for new (and perhaps older) Parkies to get off the couch and get moving.

You write honestly about the challenges presented individually and as a couple. No gloss, no rainbows, no skirting the truth, no promises, except those that can be realized by one's own hard work, belief, and persistence in the company of others."

Bob Nolte,
Retired Educator, West Hartford, CT

●

"Absolutely superb book ... concise, beautifully written ... engaging story. Never give up!

Bob Cline, M.D.,
Ocala cardiovascular surgeon, past president of the Florida Medical Association

●

"Essential reading for any family with Parkinson's."

David Lawrence, Jr.
Retired Publisher, The Miami Herald

COUNTERPUNCH:
DUKING IT OUT WITH
PARKINSON'S

Gil Thelen *with*
C. Struby Thelen

The information in this book is intended to be helpful and inspirational and does not replace professional medical or legal advice in dealing with Parkinson's. The authors' intent is to help Parkies and their care partners take aggressive action to stay upright, moving, productive, and to NOT be a victim to PD. Any use of the advice herein is at the reader's/your discretion. The authors and publisher assume no direct or indirect responsibility or liability for your actions.

Excerpt(s) from A GENERAL THEORY OF LOVE by Thomas Lewis, Richard Lannon and Fariborz Amini, copyright © 2002 by Thomas Lewis, Richard Lannon and Fariborz Amini, used by permission of Random House, an imprint and division of Penguin Random House LLC. All rights reserved. Any third party use of this material, outside of this publication, is prohibited. Interested parties must apply directly to Penguin Random House LLC for permission.

Because of the dynamic nature of the internet, any links or web addresses contained in this book may have changed since Counterpunch's publication or since publication of the original material cited.

Print ISBN: 978-1-54394-541-6

eBook ISBN: 978-1-54394-542-3

DEDICATION

Dedicated to the late Gerard Herrero
and his widow Valerie, a passionate and tireless battler
for the welfare of people with Parkinson's.
Gerard, a quick-witted, loving man
with a mischievous twinkle in his eyes,
fought Parkinson's at every turn.
He never, ever, gave in or gave up;
never failed to rise from the mat, blow after blow inflicted
by the enigmatic Parkinson's invader
to his central nervous system.

CONTENTS

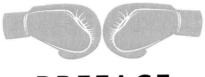

PREFACE

You are stunned to hear you have Parkinson's (PD).

You are a certified Person With Parkinson's (PWP), or a Parkie, as I prefer to be called.

Your options are just two: 1. Take to the couch (or recliner) and let the Beast grind you down one bodily system at a time. 2. Get vertical, get moving, and engage the Beast at every step of your journey. Counterpunch the bastard. Dizzy him with metaphorical jabs, hooks, and uppercuts. Take back a portion of the ground he has gained from you.

That's it. A stark, binary decision. Fight or melt away.

This Call To Action is about my choice of Option 2.

I will try to answer the two questions I get most often.

"I've just been diagnosed with Parkinson's. What will happen to me?"

"What's it like having Parkinson's?"

I can offer no easy answer to either, but I will address both.

PD is an ultimately unknowable condition. Each case is unique to the person. Men are 50% more affected than women. Even the numbers are approximations. One million cases in the U.S. Seven million worldwide. Fifty thousand new cases a year in the U.S. Second most common neurological disorder after Alzheimer's.

One million cases in a nation of more than 320 million persons. A mere drop in the bucket, right? High public awareness of PD suggests otherwise.

I speak often to civic organizations about PD. I invariably ask, "How many of you know someone with PD?" Routinely, more than a third of the group raises their hands. In one group, 100% of the hands went up.

What about the question, "What will a PD diagnosis mean in my life?" The best answer I can give is "everything."

My stab on the what's-it-like question is this: every day with PD is different. Funky, sometimes. Apathetic, others. Disorganized, frequently. Sometimes, even the old "normal."

Rarely is there a reason to explain the difference, except one: **stress**. The more stress, the greater the intensity and number of symptoms. Less stress, fewer and milder symptoms.

I will share my experience since diagnosis in 2014 at age 75. I was a semi-retired journalist, executive director of the Florida Society of News Editors, and part-time college professor in Tampa, FL.

I retired in 2006 as president and publisher of the then-thriving *Tampa Tribune* (now shuttered). Previously I was executive editor of *The State* newspaper (Columbia, SC) and editor of *The Sun News* (Myrtle Beach, SC). Before that, I was a senior editor of *The Charlotte Observer* and a Washington correspondent for 12 years. At diagnosis, I was Clendinen Professor of critical writing at the School of Mass Communications, University of South Florida (USF).

My university was Duke (history major and pre-med). Intending to be a physician, I successfully completed two years of classes at Cornell University Medical College. I decided instead to become a health and medicine reporter, which became my specialty as a Washington correspondent. (Associated Press, Consumer Reports, Chicago Daily News)

It was impossible to imagine then how my medical training and writing would sharpen my sparring with PD 50 years later.

I chronicle my PD journey on my blog www.shufflingeditor.com. The shuffling refers to my foot-dragging that kicks up scatter rugs.

"Counterpunch" makes no effort to be encyclopedic or definitive on Parkinson's. It is one man's (and his wife's) story of counterpunching the many assaults and disabilities PD has dealt me. I recount my strategies and workarounds to stay upright, moving, and productive.

My fundamental message is: Take aggressive action. Shape your future. Don't be a victim. Persevere.

I owe a huge debt of gratitude to Diane Cook, the Parkie genius who developed an enormously powerful training program that has guided me in my journey. It equips Parkies with the knowledge and mental tools to ease the symptoms of this progressive, incurable but treatable condition.

My second debt of gratitude is to the founders and practitioners of Rock Steady Boxing. It's a PD therapeutic training program that goes well beyond punching a heavy bag. The book title comes from my Rock Steady experience and being a Duke grad.

The words I live by are Love, Laugh, Hope, Pray, Persevere.

The tone of this book is meant to be informal and sometimes cheeky—like the newsroom cultures I so love. I expect you will sometimes find me venturing too far out the verbal diving board. Forgive me.

This book also serves as a guide to how Parkies and their care partners can organize at ground level to Live Well With Parkinson's, the call to action of the Davis Phinney Parkinson's Foundation.

I believe effective organization rests on a three-legged stool:

1. Informed and empowered Parkies and partners

2. Healthcare providers working in tandem to develop treatment strategies for each patient—a Parkie's individualized "Plan"

3. A local Parkinson's Center—virtual or bricks-and-mortar—where patients and partners can locate the resources they need to fulfill their individualized action plans

My foundation, Me-Over-PD (MOPD), works in two, soon to be three (Detroit), communities.

My wife Struby and I lived in Tampa for 20 years. There, we are in the final testing stage of a live database of crucial resources, including neurologists specializing in mobility diseases, physical therapists, speech therapists, occupational therapists, dietitians, and personal trainers, to name a few.

Newly diagnosed individuals will receive—for the first time anywhere—real-time, verified, actionable, and local information to assist them in navigating this mysterious condition.

In Macon, GA, where we now live, Struby and I host meetings for Parkies and care partners to discuss the nuances of PD and design action steps to improve care for all patients in Middle Georgia. We call those "Study/Action Groups."

In addition to the Study/Action Groups, I am working with Mercer University's medical school to improve Parkinson's awareness among current and future physicians.

Struby has assembled a list of local resources recommended by patients and care partners to assist Parkies in carrying out their individual wellness plans. We refer to it as "MOPD Lite."

I hope the experiences my wife and I recount will give fellow Parkies and their care partners a few useful tools to counterpunch PD, a wicked condition indeed.

Gil Thelen
Macon, GA
August 2018

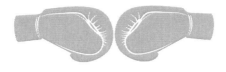

CHAPTER 1:

"It Won't Kill You"

The physician assistant (PA) studied my walk. My right arm swing was out of sync with my left. Right was lower.

Case closed.

"It appears to be Parkinson's," she said, almost cheerfully. "The good news is it's treatable. And it won't kill you. Something else will.

"The bad news is Parkinson's is progressive and incurable."

I heard those carefully chosen words on an early spring day in 2014. The exact date I don't remember.

Not remembering diagnosis day is quite unusual among Parkies. For most, it's a red-letter day, the day their lives changed forever.

Me?

I was more relieved than shocked at the news. Finally, I had an answer for the bedeviling symptoms that had been mounting since 2006: depression, extreme fatigue, leathery fingers, violent night-mares acted out at my wife's expense.

In one vivid dream, I was a soldier in World War I. Germans were attacking my position. I hurled myself down an embankment, arms flailing. One arm, in real time, struck my wife.

At other times dreams threw me out of bed, knocking over and breaking the bedside table and lamp and cutting my forehead on the table edge. (The cut was quite close to my eye, and blood still stains the carpet.)

Tell your internist about the dreams and their increasing frequency, my wife Struby said. "I am worried."

Just old-man stuff, I thought to myself. No way to stop them. Waste of time to bother a busy doctor with that.

Wrong call.

Had I messaged my internist Elizabeth Warner about the dreams, the PD diagnosis could have come months earlier and treatment started sooner. (The action-filled dreams, REM sleep disorder, are a hallmark of PD.)

In retrospect, I saw that some physical deterioration I had experienced was due to Lewy Body (see Glossary for definition) damage, not normal aging.

I had difficulty throwing a baseball. I was progressively losing distance on the golf course.

A 240-yard drive in 2010 limped to 180 yards in 2015. I hung up my golf shoes and clubs that year after playing passionately for 55 years. I could no longer swing a club and maintain balance. (I returned to the game in late 2017 after intense training and exercise restored much of my lost balance and equilibrium.)

There were behavioral changes. I had uncharacteristically withdrawn from faculty friends at USF in the months before diagnosis. Depression was squashing my normal exuberance.

My classroom energy was lower. I loved coaching and teaching. But some days I shortened class to fit what energy I had.

Rewinding to the time before diagnosis, my internist and her colleagues continued to search for answers to my case.

Vitamin B-12 deficiency perhaps? Nope. Monthly B-12 injections didn't do much.

The odd leathery feeling in my hands sent me to a neurologist, referred by the internist. B-12 deficiency can cause peripheral nerve damage. The peripheral test for damage was negative.

But the PA's test of my balance, muscle tone and walk revealed the true malefactor. It was PD killing off dopamine-producing neurons in my brain.

Oddly enough, symptoms often don't appear until 60% to 80% of the dopamine neurons are dead.

Yet the PA's diagnosis was tentative. No blood or other routine tests can identify PD beyond any doubt.

Proof of diagnosis is considered to be significant symptom improvement after adjusting to the drug carbidopa-levodopa (Sinemet). The drug is commonly called the "Gold Standard" for treating PD.

The PA sketched instructions on paper for phasing in the medication over a month. See the doctor in three months, she said, making the appointment.

That was it.

No counseling about managing the condition. No mention of what to tell or not tell loved ones, friends, or employer. No pamphlets explaining Parkinson's. No advice about trustworthy information, online and off. No mention of support groups to join.

I was figuratively shown the door, alone in the parking lot with the malady that would shape the rest of my days. The parking lot was part of a university medical center designated a National Center of Excellence for PD care.

Compared to most newly diagnosed Parkies, I was fortunate. I had medical training. I was a reporter trained to seek validated, reliable information. I had been an editor-in-chief of large newsrooms, accustomed to aggressively making and carrying out complicated plans.

What if I had none of those experiences? I shudder at the thought.

●   ●   ●

Lessons Learned

No system of care exists if you have Parkinson's, unless your treatment is from an extremely small handful of highly specialized and patient-centered institutions.

It's all on you. You live by your ingenuity and perseverance. Good luck. Indeed.

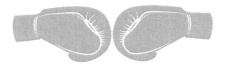

CHAPTER 2:

Researching My Malady

Malady identified. Parkinson's. Time to report the medical story of my life.

I sought accurate, verified, and crystal clear information: standard ingredients of good journalism.

I knew the playing field.

Google and the internet were first. The information there was voluminous, disjointed, and often of questionable origin and intent, commercial or otherwise.

Next, the websites of the three major foundations focused on PD: Davis Phinney Foundation for Parkinson's, Michael J. Fox Foundation, and Parkinson's Foundation.

The information was straightforward and mostly well organized. My research found the sites trustworthy, accurate, and reliable.

Each overlaps with the others but is somewhat specialized. Fox focuses on drug research. Davis Phinney has exercise and wellness as its niche. The Parkinson's Foundation is known for patient education and advocacy.

My friend Kirk Hall, a Parkie, has assembled a comprehensive list of information available on leading sites. It appears on his website www.shakypawsgrampa.com and is listed at the conclusion of this chapter. It is a wise compilation and deserves widespread attention.

He has devoted much of his great energy and intelligence to designing new care systems for PWP. I write more about Kirk's work in Chapter 11.

One of Kirk's recommendations deserves special note: the invaluable PF publication *Parkinson's Disease Q&A Seventh Edition (Q&A)*.

The most complete PD compendium is the Davis Phinney's *Every Victory Counts (EVC)*.

I give *Q&A* and *EVC* to newly diagnosed Parkies I meet. *EVC* is available free to download or order at www.davis-phinneyfoundation.org/resources/every-victory-counts-2017/. Order or download the *Q&A* free at www.parkinson.org/pd-library/books/Q-and-A-Seventh-Edition.

The Davis Phinney Foundation (https://www.davis-phinneyfoundation.org/resources/worksheets-and-down-loads/), Parkinson's Foundation (http://www.parkinson.org/pd-library), American Parkinson Disease Association (https://www.apdaparkinson.org/resources-support/download-publications/), and Michael J. Fox Foundation (https://www.michaeljfox.org/foundation/publications.html?category=5&navid=newsletters-releases) have newsletters, brochures, videos, blogs, and fact sheets that can be ordered, viewed, or downloaded free.

When my initial reporting was done, I wrote a column for *The Tampa Tribune*. Excerpts follow:

It's a snowflake condition. Just like a snowflake, each of us is unique and so is our Parkinson's. Do not assume your condition will look like someone else's.

Some symptoms are invisible. Because many of us associate Parkinson's with movement symptoms, we may ignore signs of depression, fatigue, constipation, or sleep problems (especially acting-out nightmares). In recent years the medical field has recognized such symptoms are part of the condition. If you experience them, tell your doctor so they can be diagnosed and treated for what they really represent.

[See Appendix A: Bodily Symptoms Checklist]

A Parkinson's specialist is invaluable. Many of us see a general neurologist for our care without realizing we might benefit from seeing a movement disorder specialist (MDS). An MDS is a neurologist who has undergone two years of additional training. An MDS can help us to better manage the condition and stay current on research and clinical trials.

Staying active is essential. Parkinson's may affect our movement, but staying active can help in the long run. Research shows that intensive, sustained exercise (such as boxing, tai chi, Hatha yoga, interval cycling) can ease symptoms, combat fatigue, and reduce stress. Regular daily activity (going for walks, doing the laundry) can also help improve life with Parkinson's.

We can benefit from complementary care. In addition to medications, we can benefit from physical, speech, and occupational therapy; the knowledge of nutritionists and psychotherapists; and, the wisdom and moxie of social workers. Putting together a care team of these professionals early on can pay off for years to come. Due to the fragmentation of PD care delivery, however, it takes considerable effort to assemble that team.

All support groups are not created equal. Support groups have different constituencies (young/elderly onset, newly diagnosed), different energy levels, different ambitions, and agendas. Shop widely before you choose—or join several.

Localized information is often scarce. Patients want close-to-home answers. Where do I locate the physical therapy that doctors often suggest? How do I find a personal trainer who specializes in PD? Who can help me make my home safe from falls? Where do I enroll in recommended tai chi, spinning, or boxing classes? In most locales, answers to those and dozens more local questions cannot be found in one place. National PD organizations offer effective national advice but can only do so much at the granular, local level.

We can live well. Most importantly, I learned it is not only possible to corral the condition but essential to do so. Never, never give in to the condition or lose hope. Significant cognitive decline and dementia are worrisome (but not inevitable) accomplices to PD neuromuscular difficulties.

Here's Kirk Hall's useful resource guide (links updated as of mid-2018):

Help locating a movement disorder neurologist and why this is important:

- *Michael J. Fox Foundation (MJFF): https://www.partnersinparkinsons.org/ find-movement-disorder-specialist?cid=aff_00032*

- *Parkinson's Foundation (PF): http://www. parkinson.org/expert-care/Patient-Centered-Care/ Finding-the-Right-Doctor*

Exercise information:

- *Davis Phinney Foundation (DPF): https://www. davisphinneyfoundation.org/living-well/exercise/*

- *Brian Grant Foundation (BGF): http://www.briangrant.org/ exercise/*

- *PF: http://www.parkinson.org/understanding-parkinsons/ treatment/Exercise/Neuroprotective-Benefits-of-Exercise*

Newly diagnosed information:

- *PF: http://www.parkinson.org/understanding-parkinsons/ what-is-parkinsons*

- *MJFF: https://www.michaeljfox.org/understanding-parkinsons/index.html?navid=understanding-pd*

- American Parkinson Disease Association (APDA): http://www.apdaparkinson.org/parkinsons-disease/understanding-the-basics/

Young onset information:

- APDA: http://www.apdaparkinson.org/national-young-onset-center/

- PF: http://www.parkinson.org/understanding-parkinsons/what-is-parkinsons/young-onset-parkinsons

Help locating a support group (PWP & care partner):

- PF: http://www.parkinson.org/find-help/resources-in-your-community

- APDA: http://www.apdaparkinson.org/resources-support/local-resources/

Talk directly to a person who can help:

- PF: http://www.parkinson.org/Living-with-Parkinsons/Resources-and-Support/Helpline/FAQs

- PF: http://www.parkinson.org/Living-with-Parkinsons/Resources-and-Support/Ask-the-Doctor-Forums

- MJFF: https://www.michaeljfox.org/understanding-parkinsons/ask_md.html?navid=ask-md

- ADPA: https://www.apdaparkinson.org/resources-support/ask-the-doctor/

● ● ●

Lesson Learned

Four websites provide a wealth of reliable Parkinson's information: American Parkinson Disease Association (www.apdaparkinson.org), Davis Phinney Foundation for Parkinson's (www.davisphinneyfoundation.org), Michael J. Fox Foundation (www.michaeljfox.org), and Parkinson's Foundation (www.parkinson.org).

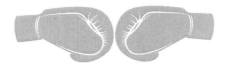

CHAPTER 3:

Had Tom Graboys Been A Neurologist

After writing *The Tampa Tribune* column, I encountered two books that changed my understanding of PD. Both challenged me to serve fellow Parkies more vigorously and effectively.

One is the autobiography of the late Thomas Graboys, MD. The other is the provocative and authoritative masterwork of journalist and Parkie Jon Palfreman.

Graboys was a beloved Boston cardiologist who struggled for many years with dementia connected to his Parkinson's. He famously wrote a book, *Life in the Balance: A Physician's Memoir of Life, Love, and Loss with Parkinson's Disease and Dementia*. It bared his innermost thoughts and emotions about the feel and look of advancing Parkinson's and dementia.

I imagined how Graboys, a master at patient care, would break the news of a Parkinson's diagnosis if he were a neurologist and not a cardiologist.

All of us end up in the neurologist's office with a variety of seemingly unrelated problems. That's one of the many things that make PD so frustrating.

When the doctor's verdict is rendered—Parkinson's—it is the day many will never forget. For some like me, there is a sense of relief that the accumulating symptoms have a cause and a name. For others, the reaction is terror, shock, and confusion.

We ask, "What does this mean for us?" A brusque answer one person received was: "Your symptoms will only get worse." In my case, the answer was: "At your age of 75, something else will kill you first." Few receive information beyond the diagnosis that day.

Commonly, we leave the doctor's office with a pill prescription and instructions to return in three months. We are on our own. We get no literature explaining what Parkinson's is, what we can do about it, and what our future holds. What if Tom Graboys had been the one delivering the news?

He would have taken the time to give us a short explanation of the condition, encouragement about the therapies available to treat it, and some information about the importance of exercise and diet.

He would have given us a set of instructions about exactly where on the internet we could find reliable information, where and what specific exercises we should seek, and information about support groups in our area. He would tell us that patients who do well with Parkinson's don't let it own them—they own and control it. "You don't have to do this alone," he would say.

Graboys would not have done this from behind his desk but sitting close to us in a reassuring manner. He would have written down on a piece of his stationery his home phone number and told us to call anytime we needed help. He would not have said to return in three months, but in one month. At that second meeting, we would discuss what we had read and the questions we had.

Graboys also would explain at that second meeting that there was a Parkinson's center to join. It would provide educational seminars, special programs for caregivers, and recommendations on finding physical and other therapists. He would work closely with the center to see that our care plan was carried out.

The Graboys approach would reduce our anxieties and provide an organizational anchor.

Graboys would write out the medications he was recommending and what they were for. He would ask us what we thought was a reasonable exercise regimen. Dietary and other lifestyle changes would be discussed to help us enhance our life. He would call those elements our *plan.*

It was the "contract" between Graboys and patient that, if adhered to, would help ensure a positive outcome. And because the plan was personal to each patient, it was more likely to be honored.

Just leaving the office with a plan inspired hope because the message was implicit that we could do things to take control of our illness.

Indeed, while 300 words may have been on that page, there really was just one: **hope**. The written plan inspired hope that by following instructions we could enhance our chances of living out a fairly normal life.

The second book is Jon Palfreman's *Brain Storms: The Race To Unlock The Mysteries of Parkinson's Disease.*

Palfreman is an experienced journalist and educator who was diagnosed in 2011. He is best known for his documentary PBS work on Frontline and NOVA.

In his book you meet a skilled dancer, Pamela Quinn, who after developing PD found ways to retrain her brain functions so she could still dance gracefully.

Writes Palfreman: "*... Quinn is certainly an outlier, with a slowly progressing form of the disease. But we can all learn from her. Her wisdom exhorts Parkies to keep active, to mindfully circumvent gait and balance issues.*"

As Quinn puts it, " 'We must treat the mind as a muscle; it needs to be strengthened and made flexible just as much as our legs and core muscles.' "

Palfreman argues persuasively that the classic symptoms of PD—rigidity, slowness, and balance problems—may be what he calls "… the tip of a clinical iceberg. It now seems that Parkinson's disease takes hold of an individual decades before any tremors appear and continues wreaking damage throughout the brain until the end of life. …"

A patient's symptoms can be far ranging, well beyond the classic neuromuscular ones. Palfreman writes:

"In the light of this evidence, many neuroscientists are lobbying to rebrand Parkinson's disease from a motor disorder to a whole-body condition, involving an enormous number of signs, symptoms, and complaints.

"These include not only the classic features—such as bradykinesia, tremor, rigidity, postural instability, stooped posture, shuffling gait, freezing of gait, dystonia, facial masking, small handwriting, dysarthria (problems with articulation), dysphagia (trouble swallowing), oily skin, bladder problems, pain, constipation, and loss of smell—but a growing list of other problems as well.

"People with Parkinson's experience neuropsychiatric symptoms such as depression, anxiety, hallucinations, cognitive impairment, and impulse control disorder (the last caused by dopamine agonists). They suffer from a whole host of sleep-related disorders—including REM sleep behavior disorder, excessive daytime sleepiness, restless legs syndrome, insomnia, and disordered breathing while sleeping. …"

Palfreman pulls no punches in describing PD's trajectory.

"… people with Parkinson's progressively lose core pieces of themselves. We forget how to walk. Our arm muscles get weaker. Our movements slow down. Our hands fumble simple fine-motor tasks like buttoning a shirt or balancing spaghetti on a fork. Our *faces no longer express emotions. Our voices lose volume and clarity. Our minds, in time, may lose their sharpness ... and more."*

The "more" varies widely from patient to patient. Some lose the sense of smell. Some shuffle instead of stride, freeze in place as they try passing through a doorway. Some drool. Some have all the symptoms, others just a few. Some are dramatically helped by the drug regimen prescribed, others continue to struggle as the regimen gets tweaked.

Palfreman fingers the alpha-synuclein protein as the major culprit, writing: *"I find the notion that the disabling symptoms of Parkinson's disease that I and other Parkies experience are caused by toxic species of alpha-synuclein spreading prion-like* [think Mad Cow Disease] *throughout the brain to be a very powerful one indeed. In a story with many setbacks, this body of research gives me genuine hope, for it suggests that in theory chemical interventions to break up and destroy the misfolded protein aggregates might help slow, stop, or reverse Parkinson's. If given early enough, such treatment might even prevent the disease from ever reaching clinical significance."*

[See Appendix B: The Rogue Protein Behind Parkinson's Disease May Also Protect Your Gut]

Writing in the *New York Times*, Palfreman said:

"Here's the theory scientists have come up with: Sometimes good proteins go bad. For multiple reasons (like genes, environment and age) proteins can 'misfold' and stick to other proteins. When proteins do this, they can become toxic, capable of jumping from cell to cell, causing other alpha-synuclein proteins to do the same and potentially killing neurons (especially dopamine-producing ones) in their wake. This process is not confined to Parkinson's disease. ..."

An intriguing hypothesis Palfreman offers is that until recently, human beings rarely lived beyond their middle years. Could it be, he asks, that aging cells lose their ability to produce healthy alpha-synuclein?

In *Brain Storms*, Palfreman quotes Cambridge University protein chemist Christopher Dobson as saying nature requires *"… that we live long enough to pass on our genes to our offspring, but it doesn't really care after that. 'And so it's evolved proteins that are stable enough and protected well enough by cellular defense mechanisms to last forty, fifty, or sixty years, but there's not much margin of safety.' "*

Palfreman concludes that he thinks the following four issues, in particular, are important for the Parkinson's community.

1. Improved delivery of levodopa to the brain: Less than 10% of a typical dosage actually reaches the brain due to the competition with other proteins to cross the blood-brain barrier.

2. The placebo effect: This is where a patient is given a dummy medication in a clinical trial of some other medication yet feels symptomatic relief.

Medicine Net defines the placebo response this way: *"A remarkable phenomenon in which a placebo—a fake treatment, an inactive substance like sugar, distilled water, or saline solution—can sometimes improve a patient's condition simply because the person has the expectation that it will be helpful. …"*

1. Recognizing the importance of non-motor symptoms such as cognition, sleep disorder, pain, and depression.

2. The need to develop personalized medicine: Palfreman defines this as a *"… collaborative culture of care where 'specialized professionals and engaged patients work together to try to achieve optimal outcomes.' "*

Personalized medicine intrigues me. An example is Parkinson Place in Sarasota, FL. It is an integrated facility with education, social activity, exercise, and counseling for people in different stages of their condition. It involves teams of providers such as a neurologist, therapist, psychologist, and legal experts.

I write about two other examples of personalized medicine in Chapters 10 and 11.

●   ●   ●

Lessons Learned

Parkinson's can involve many bodily functions, making it in all likelihood a systemic condition.

End-stage PD can be stark but must be faced to plan properly your remaining life.

Models exist for engaging patients in improving their care and increasing their odds of living well with Parkinson's.

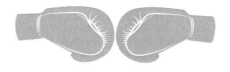

CHAPTER 4.

Parkinson's Lightning Strike

You look terrific!"

I get that, or a variant, from clued-in friends.

Mini-me wants to say: "Expect to see me drooling in a wheelchair?" Or, "Surprised that I'm still vertical?"

Mini-me suppressed.

Instead, "I am a deceptively lustrous used car—great looking, but a mess under the hood."

My visible symptoms are modest. Mild tremor in my right hand. Slower, shuffling walk. Careful steps due to balance and equilibrium issues.

Inside lie the big problems. At their untreated worst they include: hot flashes (yes, my chuckling female friends), busted gyroscope, marathon peeing (up to three times an hour), spastic bladder, non-firing colon, buckets of drinking water a day. Loss of feeling in both hands, especially the right.

I am a poster boy for PD Non-Motor Symptoms, a catch-all for big, big problems.

Let Dr. David E. Riley explain those in some detail. He has been a guest blogger on my site www.shufflingeditor.com.

Riley, an MDS neurologist, has an integrated PD patient care center in Cleveland, OH. He modeled it after Parkinson Place in Sarasota.

Dr. Riley, the floor is yours.

"One of the most important developments in the study of Parkinson's disease in the last 25 years has been recognition of its non-motor complications. Neurologists still diagnose PD by identifying the traditional motor manifestations (tremor, slowness, soft voice, small handwriting, etc.), but they have come to realize that, for many people with PD, non-motor symptoms can become even more of a problem."

Non-motor manifestations fall into four categories: *"... cognitive and psychiatric complications, autonomic nervous system disturbances, sensory abnormalities, and sleep disorders. Each ... comprises ... problems, although they are often interrelated."*

"Cognitive" refers to higher-order functions of the nervous system such as thinking, processing, decision-making, memory, communication.

"Dementia" is *"... a loss of more than one of these* [cognitive] *capacities. People with PD are at high risk of dementia. It is an ominous development ..."* producing its own problems and *"... limits our ability to treat other manifestations of PD."*

"Psychiatric" *"... refers to a group of disorders. ..."* Foremost *"... is depression, which will affect about 50% of people with PD. ..."* Depression *"... often occurs before people even know they have PD, and... may precede motor symptoms by many years. ..."*

It's not depression resulting from the realization you have PD. That's a different matter.

"... Other common psychiatric complications are hallucinations, illusions, and delusions, which result from an interaction between the brain disease and the medications people take.

"Psychiatric manifestations of PD are frequently considered alongside cognitive complications because they often coexist. Both are major sources of care-partner/caregiver stress."

The autonomic (involuntary) nervous system functions automatically, outside our control. We do control our voluntary nervous system. We determine its actions, such as cross your legs or scratch that itch.

"... Major responsibilities of the autonomic nervous system include regulation of blood pressure and heart rate, bladder and sexual function, digestive and bowel function, and control of perspiration and body temperature. PD potentially disrupts all these.

"The most common symptom of autonomic impairment is constipation. Two autonomic problems that seem to cause the most disability are an inability to maintain blood pressure, resulting in lightheadedness and fainting, and loss of bladder control.

"Sensory disturbances are an underappreciated aspect of PD. They include the loss of smell ..." and restless legs syndrome.

"Sleep disorders in PD ... include insomnia, excessive daytime sleepiness, and a ... tendency to act out one's dreams, known as REM-sleep behavior disorder."

REM disorder is "... a major tool of researchers because of its striking ability to predict the development of PD and related disorders many years ..." before diagnosis.

"Virtually all people with PD report some non-motor symptoms, but the number and types vary tremendously from person to person. This explains why no two people experience PD in exactly the same way. ...

"People with PD should ..." not assume that a particular non-motor manifestation "... will necessarily happen to them or ..." expect "... that medications will affect them in the same way as someone else. I like to compare this variability of PD to a salad bar. Even though everyone comes away with a salad, the number and assortment of ingredients is never the same for any two people.

"Non-motor manifestations ..." account "... for much of the disability and loss of quality of life. ... For many, non-motor *symptoms represent their greatest challenge. ..."* Those with PD should discuss any non-motor symptom with their doctors.

One other potentially dangerous, non-motor manifestation is visuospatial disorder. Visuospatial processing is the ability to tell where objects are in space. That includes your own body parts. It also involves being able to tell how far objects are from you and from each other. Those deficits link to driving problems like lane drifting, driving too close to other cars, hitting curbs and crooked parking.

Now about my PD lightning strike.

I had been doing fine until 30 months after diagnosis. Typical were Rock Steady Boxing three times a week, spinning twice a week, and deep involvement with my newspaper, church, and PD advocacy work.

In what seemed an instant, everything changed.

I was dizzy, wobbly on my feet, afraid of falling. I couldn't quench my thirst. I was peeing three times an hour. No energy. Withdrawn.

The lightning struck hard while my wife Struby and I traveled to the Carolinas, visiting friends and family. I was a mess on the trip home.

I wasn't judging distances properly, made a sloppy left turn and almost ran off the road.

Half an hour later, Struby screamed and grabbed the steering wheel of our Mazda CX9. I had dozed off.

It was an excruciating drive on I-77, I-26, I-95, I-10, and I-75. I needed every rest stop. Some were even too far apart. I peed in my shoes twice on the 16-hour trip, normally nine hours.

Our marriage, quite understandably, took a hit. It needed work to manage this new development. Lots of work.

My autonomic nervous system (ANS) was shot full of holes. Machine-gunned, if you will.

Urinary system kaput. Temperature regulation out of control (those hot flashes). Balance and equilibrium so wasted that I could no longer box or spin. I feared falling. I was apathetic and fatigued much of every day.

PD's hard right put me on the canvas, at least temporarily.

I grabbed the ring's ropes and metaphorically staggered to my feet. It was time to land some punches against the malady in its advance. (A progressive condition, which PD is, "advances.")

Doctors first.

I tried to arrange a conference call with my neurologist (MDS) joining my internist, Lucy Guerra, in a three-way conversation.

No sale with my MDS. Not interested in an interdisciplinary medical intervention (neurology and internal medicine working as a single team on my behalf).

We moved forward separately.

Struby and I met with my MDS. He said the lightning strike was simply PD progressing. He offered no remedies for the kidney, temperature, and balance/equilibrium disasters.

In effect, his message was: Roll with the punches. That's life with PD, your unwelcome tenant.

Next, Struby and I met with internist Guerra. She agreed with the "progressing" diagnosis of our MDS, but she was willing to take on my disaster sites with specific medications. She referred me to a urologist for a bladder work-up.

Between the two I got some relief from my worst symptoms. The medications from Guerra and urologist Jorge Lockhart worked.

I called my college fraternity brother, David Paulson, asking his advice. Paulson is a retired urologist living in Florida. He served many years as head of urology at the Duke University Medical Center.

I needed additional help, and he recommended Duke or the University of Florida (UF).

I chose UF and encountered the remarkable Michael Okun, M.D. for the second time. We had spoken briefly at the World

Parkinson's Congress several months earlier. The topics then were similar family names and a friend in common.

Okun's UF bio says this:

Okun is the "...**Administrative Director and Co-director of the Center for Movement Disorders and Neurorestoration.** *The center has over 40 interdisciplinary faculty members from 10 UF departments and 6 colleges.*

"Dr. Okun has championed interdisciplinary care both at UF and in his role as the **National Medical Director** *for the Parkinson's Foundation. ... Okun was a co-founder of the Center for Movement Disorders and Neurorestoration and has implemented its completely patient-centric approach to care."*

Okun has written several books, the best-known being *Parkinson's Treatment: 10 Secrets to a Happier Life.*

I emailed Okun about receiving care from his team. He responded within minutes. "Yes. Come on up to Gainesville. We'll set up your intake examination within a few weeks."

Okun's passion for patient care stunned me. I immediately thought of David Lawrence Jr., my customer-obsessed boss at *The Charlotte Observer.* Both men put patients/customers first and demanded their team do likewise.

Okun shared the patient-first philosophy of Tom Graboys, the Boston cardiologist I wrote about in Chapter 3.

My second counterpunch was a broader mobilization of my care team.

I turned to two other remarkable practitioners on my care team: Personal trainer Jordan Brannon and physical therapist (PT) Dr. Matt Lazinski.

Brannon, while only in her early 20s, directs her family-owned Rock Steady Boxing franchise in the Tampa Bay area. She is skillful, confident, and wise well beyond her years.

Lazinski, once a top intercollegiate tennis player, earned a doctorate in physical therapy. He talks and moves nonstop in the action area he shares with other USF PTs.

Brannon and Lazinski teamed to restore much of my balance and equilibrium.

Thanks to them I resumed my Rock Steady Boxing and spinning classes.

I am convinced Brannon and Lazinski helped me establish new brain pathways to replace those destroyed in the lightning strike. (Remember the story of the dancer who recovered her skills in Jon Palreman's book *Brain Storms*.)

That recovery process is "neuroplasticity." I will write more about it in Chapter 5. It is a vital tool when sparring with PD.

●   ●   ●

Lessons Learned

Parkinson's non-motor manifestations can progress instantly and brutally, taking you to your knees.

You can recover much lost ground through neurorestoration (restoration of a brain function through the development of new neurons and/or new neural pathways).

Tightly coordinated medical care is essential for recovery.

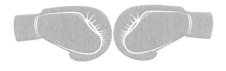

CHAPTER 5:

The Stress Villain

"**G**od has abandoned me," I said.

"Never," The Rev. Jim Harnish answered. "Not you. Not any-one. Never."

Two years later I had a conversation that oddly connected to the one with Jim.

"Please, nurse, help me fill out this form," I said. "I cannot do it myself. I can no longer write legibly."

Stress connects the two conversations. Stress big and small. Existential stress and mundane stress. God and handwriting.

Stress is this Parkie's supreme challenge. It brings on or ampli-fies other symptoms. It accelerates PD's relentless march to dimin-ish my powers and my sense of control.

Nothing in my life is natural and easy any longer: not walking, talking, eating, peeing, defecating, bathing, dressing, sleeping, driving, planning, remembering, making love, making do.

Parkinson's blows demand retaliation: ankle-biting insurrec-tions. I call them my *workarounds*—ploys that take back some lost ground.

What were my major stresses, outside the obvious one of having PD?

My daily energy was less. So why was I still investing in people and activities that were peripheral to the needs of my new life? I was hanging on to responsibilities from my pre-Parkinson's life.

I have an emotionally demanding loved one who has barraged me with countless and endless phone calls for decades. I did not cut off the calls.

Now there's a boundary about when and how long I will talk. When the time I allot is up, I end the call.

I also decided to stop wasting time with people who do not challenge, nourish, or really matter to me.

Hear the words from *"The Valuable Time of Maturity"* by Mario de Andrade, a Brazilian poet, novelist, musicologist, art historian, and photographer:

"I want to live among human people, very human. People who can laugh at their mistakes. ... Who do not run away from their responsibilities. Who defend human dignity. Who do not want anything else but walk along with truth, righteousness, honesty and integrity.

"The essential thing is what makes life worthwhile. I want to surround myself with people who can touch the hearts of others. People who, despite the hard knocks of life, grew up with a soft touch in their soul.

"Yes, I am in a hurry. So that I can live with the intensity, which only maturity can give me. ...

"My goal is to reach the end satisfied and at peace with my loved ones and my conscience. ..."

It was time to cut away *my* clutter and focus my agenda.

I chose two commitments: advocacy for Parkinson's patients and advocacy for the betterment of my community.

I take very seriously my Tampa church's activist directive of "Making God's Love Real." I enlisted in the effort to start a downtown out-reach ministry, The Portico.

Tampa's Hyde Park Methodist senior minister, Magrey deVega, describes The Portico this way: "It takes the DNA of this church and expresses it in a worship style that is participatory, spontaneous and organic, with weekly communion and quiet moments of meditation. It places Hyde Park on the front porch of spiritually seeking individuals who are looking for a community to converse, connect and help change the (larger) community."

I extended my Rotary pledge of "Service Above Self" by starting a Meals On Wheels route for the club.

I competed to make Tampa a test site for the powerful PD SELF (Self-Efficacy Learning Forum) patient empowerment program. We won. (I write much more about PD SELF in Chapter 10).

I promised to share my ankle biter retaliations for Parkinson's nasty punches. I list the infirmities, then my counter jabs called workarounds.

Memory: I have *ultra*-short-term memory problems. Where are the keys? Cell phone? Cigar lighter? Remembering my plan for the day usually still works.

Workarounds: Everything has its designated bag. Keys, wallet, reading glasses, pill case, business cards in my small, leather "Boy Bag." Boy Bag goes inside my leather shoulder bag/purse—my "Man Bag," which also contains cigar accessories, business cards, small electronics. Man Bag goes inside my backpack. Backpack contains other bags for electronics, headphones, and cigar accessories.

I seed the house with duplicates of needed items easily misplaced: reading glasses, styluses for computer screens, pens, and pencils. Consider the clutter necessary, please Dear Wife.

Clothes: I gained 50 pounds and pee much more frequently.

Workarounds: Buy waist expanders for too-small pants. Buy new pants with elastic waistbands for quick exits. Wear exercise pants for the same reason.

For car trips consider pants two sizes too large and adult diapers. Pride is a luxury with PD. To avoid morning choke-up on what to wear, set clothes out the day before—when your head is clear and dopamine is "on."

Get a 36-inch shoehorn. Takes the muscle strain out of putting on shoes.

[See Appendix C: Bow Ties Pummel Parkinson's]

Loss of feeling in fingers: Mine is 95% gone in my once-dominant right hand; 80% gone in the left.

Workarounds: I am training my left hand to be dominant—eating utensils, cup holding, stylus use. (Neuroplasticity, neurorestoration at work.)

Use only cups and glasses with handles to avoid "dropsies." Eat shamelessly with a spoon where a fork used to serve.

Emotional volatility: "Emotional incontinence," in a Parkie friend's unforgettable rendering.

Workaround: Think twice (maybe 10 times) before acting on impulse (binge shopping, overeating, gambling, etc.). One of my former agonists gave me a wandering eye, to my wife's chagrin. That agonist is very much gone.

Multi-tasking kaput: I can no longer perform multiple tasks at once.

Workaround: KISS (Keep It Simple, Stupid) principle always. Rely on care partner for help.

Bradykinesia (slow movements) and **bradyphrenia** (slow mental processing): Life in the slow lane. Slow walking. Slow talking. Slow thinking.

Workaround: Add 30 minutes (or more) to the time of a planned task (packing for trip, gym date, doctor visit).

Balance: Tipsy walking.

Workaround: Forget a cane or walker; use walking sticks for balance. Sexy and pleasantly eye-catching ("Cross-country skiing in Florida! How neat," was a reaction I received.) Use shopping carts in all stores to steady balance.

Bed: Having trouble turning over in bed or getting out of bed.

Workarounds: Satiny pajamas or silk sheets make it easier to turn over.

A bed rail can help you pull yourself up to get out of bed as well as keep you in bed if violent nightmares toss you around.

House: Add or get rid of things around the house that can trip you up or send you down.

Workarounds: Install grab bars in the shower and near the toilet. Add a bench or seat in the shower and in the closet.

Put in comfort-height toilets or booster seats. Ditch scatter rugs that constantly get tripped over.

Car: Leaving stuff in and around car.

Workarounds: Rigid discipline to **always** check roof, door locks, rear hatch, and ground around vehicle.

Open the garage door **first**.

Driving uncertainty: The **big** issue for many.

Workarounds: If feasible, get a technology-loaded car (GPS, blind spot displays, radar, and cameras everywhere); stick to the middle lane; U-turns rather than left turns into four-lane roads; care partner drives in unfamiliar areas.

Increase normal number of side-to-side and straight ahead eye sweeps to gain more information. Use computer program to increase peripheral vision. Take driving test offered by AAA.

If a physician qualifies you, get a handicapped parking mirror-hanger or license plate. Handicapped spots give you additional door-opening space and room to park straight, rather than Parkie-crooked.

Visuospatial deficits are a higher-order mental function problem in PD. Those deficits link to driving problems like lane drifting, driving too close to other cars, hitting curbs, and crooked parking. Visuospatial disruption is why I almost ran off the road after the PD lightning strike in the Carolinas.

Visuospatial issues also explain why I often bump into furniture and aim wrong in reaching to pick up objects, such as wine glasses. Bad aim can put (aargh!) red wine on the carpet.

●　　●　　●

Lessons Learned

Stress is Parkinson's ally. Reduce it to live better.
Use counterpunches to regain lost ground from PD's ravages.

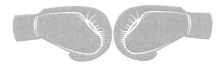

CHAPTER 6:

Exercise Is Medicine

My research convinced me exercise was essential to spar effectively with PD. But what kind and where to find it?

My first neurologist referred me to Big and Loud training at Florida Hospital Tampa. That's physical therapy for stretching tense muscles and voice modulation. I benefited but needed *Capital E* exercise.

I asked the Big and Loud PTs about that. They pointed me to tai chi exercise training.

I found tai chi a bit mannered and slow. Nice companions, but I was still searching for the *Capital E.*

Next tip was that two Tampa YMCAs were starting high-speed, spinning classes for Parkies. I began one-hour sessions twice a week spinning on stationary bikes. Felt good.

But I needed still more.

The "more" came in a newspaper article. Something called Rock Steady Boxing (RSB) was opening in a West Tampa Bay gym 45 miles from my home. Intriguing name. Worth checking out for my blog.

To see first what RSB was like, I went to the website www. rocksteadyboxing.org/videos/ and opened the YouTube video "We are Rock Steady Boxing."

I needed to see RSB in person.

Gym owner Tara Schwartz pitched program benefits this way: "Studies have shown that intense forced exercise has slowed the progression of Parkinson's. Parkinson's slows the conduction of the nerve to the muscles, so everything slows down. Boxing does the absolute opposite of that. And it's a non-contact form of boxing."

Good elevator speech, Schwartz. I watched one day. Signed up and worked out the next.

Ninety intense minutes to pulsating music and demanding, disciplined but supportive instructors: "Elbows up … jab, jab, hook … chest out, stomach in … just 10 more seconds."

Schwartz's class typically has 12 to 15 participants who work out ideally at least three days a week.

Said Schwartz: "While focusing on overall fitness, strength training, reaction time, and balance, workouts include ring work, focus mitts, heavy bags, speed bags, double ended bags, jump rope, core work, calisthenics, and circuit weight training. No boxing experience is necessary, and people of all ages are invited to participate."

Sessions typically have 30 minutes of stretching exercises, 30 minutes of weight training, and 30 minutes of work on punching bags.

Until the "Lightning Strike" (Chapter 4) put me down, I made the 90-mile round trip to the Largo gym three times a week.

Rock Steady was a tonic. It returned my energy, concentration, focus, and stamina to pre-PD levels.

I also glimpsed the power that comes with the camaraderie of working a common task with close friends. I will write more about that in Chapter 10.

A growing body of research affirms how exercise improves PD symptoms, bends the condition direction in the right way and helps the brain build new neural pathways (neurogenesis) to replace functions destroyed by PD.

The Parkinson's Foundation gets it right about exercise with this summary of the literature as of 2018:

"There is a growing consensus among researchers about the short- and long-term benefits of exercise for people with PD."

Exercise can benefit in two ways:

"Symptom management. *Research has shown that exercise can improve gait, balance, tremor, flexibility, grip strength and motor coordination. Exercise such as treadmill training and biking have all been shown to benefit, as has Tai Chi and yoga. ...*

"... There is a strong consensus among physicians and physical therapists that improved mobility by exercising may improve thinking, memory and reduce risk of falls. ..."

"At this time, we know that people who exercise vigorously, for example like running or cycling, have fewer changes in their brains caused by aging. Studies in animals suggest exercise also improves PD symptoms.

"Neurologists within the Parkinson's Foundation Center of Excellence network recommend exercise to their patients and also to people who are worried about getting PD because of a family connection." One Parkinson's Outcomes Project *"... study showed that people with PD who exercised regularly for 2.5 hours per week had a smaller decline in mobility and quality of life over two years. ..."*

"The best way to see benefits is to exercise on a consistent basis. People with PD enrolled in exercise programs with durations longer than six months, regardless of exercise intensity, have shown significant gains in functional balance and mobility as compared to programs of only two-week or 10-week durations.

"When it comes to exercise and PD, greater intensity may have greater benefits. Experts recommend that people with PD, particularly young onset or those in the early stages, exercise with intensity for as long as possible as often as possible. Your doctor might

recommend an hour a day three or four times a week, but most researchers think that the more you do, the more you benefit.

"Intense exercise is exercise that raises your heart rate and makes you breathe heavily. Studies have focused on running and bicycle riding, but experts feel that other intense exercise should provide the same benefit.

"**How does exercise change the brain?** What happens in the brain to produce these visible benefits? Researchers at the University of Southern California looked at the brains of mice that had exercised under conditions parallel to a human treadmill and discovered that:

"Exercising did not affect the amount of dopamine in the brain, but the mice that exercised the brain cells were using dopamine more efficiently.

"Exercise improves efficiency by modifying the areas of the brain where dopamine signals are received—the substantia nigra and basal ganglia."

●　　●　　●

Lesson Learned

Living the "vertical" life means exercise, and plenty of it. Try the many options to find the right fit, then stick with those exercises religiously.

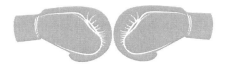

CHAPTER 7:

Parkinson's Scrambles My Thinking Life

Nothing prepared me for the Parkinson's experience "inside" me, the under-the-skin disruptions.

I prided myself, before PD, on my self-awareness. I understood my stream of consciousness and my sometimes-turbulent emotions. Or so I thought.

My Parkinson's is predominantly the non-motor kind, centering on the autonomic nervous system. That means most of my bodily functions are affected at one time or another. Dr. David Riley talked about those in Chapter 4:

"Major responsibilities of the autonomic nervous system include regulation of blood pressure and heart rate, bladder and sexual function, digestive and bowel function, and control of perspiration and body temperature. PD potentially disrupts all these.

"The most common symptom of autonomic impairment is constipation. Two autonomic problems causing the most disability are an inability to maintain blood pressure, resulting in lightheadedness and fainting, and loss of bladder control. ..."

"Sleep disorders in PD ... include insomnia, excessive daytime sleepiness, and a ... tendency to act out dreams, known as REM-sleep behavior disorder."

Awareness of inner fluctuations matters. The fluctuations often signal needed medication adjustments.

Too frequent peeing? Take a salt pill for water retention. Hot or cold flashes? Adjust my Sinemet dosage or timing intervals.

Constipation? Take an additional laxative capsule. Sleep interruptions? Increase my Trazodone dosage before bed.

Stiffness and pain in my back? Get my physical trainer to provide remedial exercise.

Heightened consciousness of inner doings led me to a closer examination of my psychological needs and behaviors.

The 800-pound gorilla was my marriage.

I met my future wife Cynthia Jane Struby at *The Charlotte Observer*, where we were both sub-editors in the late 1970s.

She went by the handle Struby, not Cynthia. "I must not look like a 'Cynthia' because no one will call me that," she has often said.

She is tall (just shy of 5'10"), statuesque, composed, smartly dressed, personable, attentive, detailed, athletic, and quite smart. The room pays attention when she enters.

Struby was a journalist from birth. Her late father, Bert Struby, was the longtime president and publisher of *The Macon Telegraph* and the now-defunct *Macon News* in Middle Georgia.

She grew to share many of his strongest traits. He was cautious, precise, quantitative, explicit, principled, devout, rule-driven, predictable, steady, and inward. What you saw was what you got.

First-child daughter started newspapering after graduation from Furman, a demanding university in South Carolina. By age 24 she had meteorically risen to managing editor of a small daily in Virginia.

It wasn't hard to fall for Struby, for all the right reasons.

We were bookends.

Me: driven, extroverted (in public settings), passionate to a fault, big-picture guy, conceptual. Myers-Briggs personality type E/INTJ.

(After PD, I added rule breaker—on occasion and when the rule is stupid. My bumper sticker reads "Obedience School Dropout.")

Struby: Deeply introverted (while seemingly not), detailed, quantitative, cautious, future-focused, rule maker, and rule follower. (If there were such a bumper sticker, hers would be "Obedience School Honor Graduate.") Her Myers-Briggs type is ISFJ.

The onset of Parkinson's dealt our marriage a staggering blow.

Over time—we later realized with outside help—we were meeting too many personal needs through others, not one another.

Struby drew support from her wide network of friends: tennis, PTA, social organizations, neighborhood, Scouts, school, professional, lacrosse parents. And her two sons.

I drew support from my profession, Rotary International, church, golf and cigar buddies.

[See Appendix D: The Tampa Humidor Trumps My Parkinson's]

PD ripped off our marital Band-Aids. Struby correctly refers to those as heavy-duty, duct-tape patches in Chapter 8.

For our marriage to survive, we had to dig deep to establish new connections and partnerships with one another.

A no-nonsense therapist pointed the way. I treasure her for her uncanny insights and pivotal guidance.

My therapeutic breakthrough came when I related my childhood to my subsequent life with women.

I love the company of women. But I harbor mistrust, always.

My mother, Violet Okonn Thelen (Vi), was a promoter of her self-importance. Always center stage. Always demanding attention and adulation. Many times she would recount triumphs such as:

- High school girlfriend of Johnny "Tarzan" Weissmuller. *Check.*

- Pioneering female Realtor in Milwaukee. *Check.*

- Owner (and grand hostess) of a successful gift shop in Richmond, VA. *Check.*

My brother Neil and I were her stagehands.

Our role was to win academic and sports honors that she would display on her massive charm bracelet. (All-Conference football and track. Phi Beta Kappa and Omicron Delta Kappa keys, to name but a few.)

Vi had a devastating way of controlling her eager-to-please and emotionally needy sons. Displease her and she would ice us emotionally, withdrawing her affection.

That experience carried forward.

I am always on guard about women pulling the emotional rug from under me.

I have never been able to fully trust any woman, including those I loved and love.

A second impediment to our marriage was my adjustment to Parkinson's unpredictability and randomness. I could not count on anything about tomorrow, including being alive to see it.

Today is all I have. Past and future matter much less than they did pre-PD.

My stream of consciousness is "in the now." I live as if today were my last on earth.

The oddity of PD symptoms draws me closer to fellow Parkies. They don't need elaborate explanation of our shared disabilities, the kind where there is no real answer to the question "Why?".

Talk is easy among Parkies. Personal ties are quite "tribal," using Davis Phinney's lovely phrase for the Parkie People in his orbit.

I increasingly had cut my wife out of my deepest engagement with Parkinson's. I thought she didn't get the randomness, the ambiguity, the non-linearity.

Struby wanted "why" answers where there were none.

Our differing needs put us on a crash course.

Struby demanded preciseness of my every thought and move. Or so I felt.

I believed she wanted to control whatever freedom was left to me after PD had taken its gigantic bite.

I remembered Tom Graboys's wonderful line about how the Beast relentlessly diminishes our powers and saps our personal control.

Three contenders pulled at my sense of control: my malady, my mate, and me. I was deeply torn.

Struby and I needed common ground, more meeting in the middle of our differing personal needs.

For me, that meant supplying the detailed information Struby needed about my thoughts and actions. It was her psychic oxygen.

I would share my daily encounters more completely and meticulously.

Struby hates "messes" in her environment. I would redouble efforts to avoid cluttering our household.

Bradykinesia is a "biggie" for us, especially with its ugly twin, bradyphrenia.

I am not any more stupid with PD, just slower in knitting my thoughts together in concrete words and coherent sentences.

Bradyphrenia results in impatience with details and diminished executive function capacities, such as multi-tasking and juggling. I have to do things one step at a time and keep them simple (KISS principle, again).

Read on in the next two chapters to learn Struby's take on managing the peculiarities of a Parkie husband. Me.

●　　●　　●

Lessons Learned

Parkinson's is an inner journey of new awareness, much of it positive. It is disastrous to cut your life partner out of details

about that journey. Communicate. Deeply communicate. More deeply communicate.

Bradyphrenia can be a bigger challenge than bradykinesia.

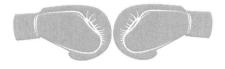

CHAPTER 8:

The Marital Duct Tape Frays

(by Struby Thelen)

"**I**f you had behaved like this when I met you, I never would have married you," I shrieked at Gil.

Shrieking is not my style. Nor is resistance to change. But Gil's adjustment to PD had me on the ropes, to borrow one of his boxing metaphors. Our marriage was coming apart. The duct-tape patches were fraying.

During 38 years of marriage we had successfully managed, *together*, several lifetimes of disruptive change. We had evolved *together*.

Our challenges had been supersized: his messy divorce and two pre-teens living with us briefly just after our 1-year wedding anniversary; eight cycles of in vitro fertilization to get pregnant; the adoption of two incredibly talented boys, each challenging in their own right; a parent with Alzheimer's living with us several years while our boys were young (about 3 and 7); the deaths of all four parents; job changes and moves; retirement and second part-time careers; full-time career to freelance career to stay-at-home-mom to PTA officer/Cub and Boy Scout leader/sports team mom to empty nester.

Our marriage could weather anything, I proudly thought.

I was **so** wrong.

We needed significant outside help.

In a soul-baring conversation 2½ years after diagnosis, Gil and I realized our marriage was more patches than a sturdy whole. It was a good thing the duct tape had been *really* strong.

The additional strain of PD was wearing our marriage's compromising patches conspicuously thin, although we both had considered the accommodations absolutely appropriate at the time.

We were fine on nuts-and-bolts decisions, such as how we wanted to arrange our legal affairs. We had laid things out with each other and an estate attorney years ago, knowing we both will die at some point. The minor tweaking and updating, given the unpredictability of PD, had been going easily.

Talking about what might lie ahead, we agreed on how to begin downsizing and where our next home should be. We educated ourselves on the variety of care options—not knowing what might be needed when—and explored retirement facilities to see where we might best fit in and be comfortable. Our #1 choice was the same location.

Since the progression of Parkinson's is so uncertain and varies from person to person, palliative—as well as end-of-life care—continues to be an open discussion between us.

Focusing on the emotional "us right now" proved to be the huge stumbling block.

We both said we wanted the marriage to work, but each of us had significant doubts. The trust that we'd shared had greatly eroded, and we realized PD and its medications were overwhelming our duct-tape patches.

How had we gotten to this dreadful place? We both jumped at the chance to add a social worker to the expanding Thelen PD Care Team to help us work through the conflicts.

Our terrific therapist quickly identified our primary challenge. For two people who were professional communicators, we were lousy at communicating deeply and openly with each other. Those are my words, not our therapist's.

We had drawn too many assumptions from each other's actions and non-actions. We had raised too few questions when we should have. When the diagnosis of PD hit, neither of us was prepared to deal with it together, as marital partners.

When Gil came home from his doctor's appointment and shared that he had Parkinson's, my first reaction was relief. Now there was a name for all those frustrating symptoms of his. Relief quickly gave way to: What exactly is Parkinson's? What does it mean for us?

I set out to learn. He did the same. But we could not find common ground to talk to each other about our findings and feelings. I thought Gil was just taking a long time to process the diagnosis. He thought I was in denial and not interested in understanding what having PD meant.

Neither of us brought up what it meant for us as a couple. We didn't talk about what each of us thought was ahead and how best to tackle PD together.

Gil didn't hesitate to say he was feeling this or that way because of Parkinson's on any given day. But he never seemed to want to talk about what it ultimately meant to him—only that he was determined to live in the moment because he did not know what the future would hold.

When I mentioned things I had read about PD, I got the distinct feeling it was either old news or did not pertain exactly to him.

He had become manic about researching his condition. Whatever I learned seemed inconsequential. He had the medical background. I did not. He had Parkinson's. I could never understand what that was like. I should not even try, his tone of voice and body language told me. PD was driving a wedge deeper into our relationship.

Looking back, we should have been able to give each other an appropriate length of time to let the diagnosis sink in and gather information about what could be ahead. Next should have been a conversation about what it meant to us, separately and together. Instead, misunderstanding whacked the wedge further into our marriage.

It took almost two years before I went to a doctor visit with my husband. I thought Gil never asked because he never wanted me there. He thought I wasn't interested in accompanying him.

He always seemed to be asserting his independence. He thought I gave higher priorities to our boys than to him and his PD issues. We were wary and stalemated.

I broke the impasse, crying that he was shutting me out of his life so completely that he didn't even want me hearing what was said at his doctor visits.

Those "shut-outs" had been coming faster and faster, I felt.

His violent dreams, which began some five or so years before diagnosis, ultimately sent him to another bedroom. Yes, I missed him greatly at night, but I now could get decent sleep. He said separate beds eased his worry about waking me up with his active dreams. So separate bedrooms were worth it from both our points of view.

His upstairs home office got traded for the neighborhood cigar bar. The house was quieter, but I did not have to worry about him tripping going up and down the stairs or have to put up with the cigar smoke and mess on the lanai. He said he enjoyed the camaraderie of his cigar-smoking friends.

Gil jumped into Parkinson's with both feet: getting trained to help others with PD, writing a blog, voraciously reading about Parkinson's, attending patient-support groups, kicking off a nine-month-long PD course, speaking at support groups and Rotary and civic club meetings, meeting with fellow Parkies to share experiences.

He had always kept busy with part-time jobs after retirement. His full calendar wasn't so new, but now he *just* wanted to be around people in the Parkie community. I was included in these new friendships and activities only when it would seem awkward for me not to be there. I still had my friends and tennis community, and surely this was a phase that would pass, I thought.

Yet I felt more and more like a prop: expected to smile and be at his side when he wanted me there. Expected to host and attend events that were important to *him*, not necessarily to *us*. I never felt needed, except when PD prevented him from doing something he had been able to handle on his own before.

In exasperation one evening I flung my glass of Kendall-Jackson Chardonnay in his face. "Just go be with your PD friends," I yelled.

I was feeling more and more like his maid: expected to cook his meals, do his laundry, cut his food, help him get dressed, put on his medication patches, clean up his cigar messes, give up my tennis at the spur of the moment to do something he thought needed to be done right then.

I felt less and less like a wife. I felt very used and unappreciated, and certainly not loved. I was quite willing to do things Gil needed me to do, as long as the full relationship was satisfying for me, too.

How had he become so cold, arrogant, autocratic, impatient, and quick to jump to conclusions? He was no longer collaborative, sharing, sensitive, caring, and loving. We were no longer married. We were co-existing—and not very amicably.

Trust had become a major issue for us. Gil began sneaking around to avoid what he said he thought would become major "justifications" or "flame-ups" to me.

When he wanted to use another brand of bath soap, for example, he purchased it himself and tried to sneak the package into the house under his coat. For me, that translated into not being able to trust him to have a simple conversation with me. Why couldn't he just tell me he wanted another brand for a change? Soap was such a minor thing. Worse, what else was he sneaking around about?

I saw his changed personality as no longer caring about our marriage or making any relationship work with others who did not operate or see things as he did. He had become hardline and unforgiving and began to cut other people out of his life besides me.

I understand a person cannot separate himself from his condition, but Gil seemed to have no room in his life for anything or anyone not associated with PD. He turned to those who agreed with him, at all hours of the day and night. I turned to my friends.

In angry desperation I said I was not going to continue to live like this. I wanted out. A divorce. "In sickness and in health" did not mean I was to put up with solely being his servant. Let him deal with whatever PD had turned him into. I was not going to spend the rest of my life in a relationship with someone who did not love or respect me.

Enter Wonderful Counselor. She was able to help us see that our issues went back further than PD, and if they were dealt with we could tackle PD together.

All those "I choose not to fight this battle now" decisions probably had been the right thing at the time, but they had gotten us in the habit of not fully sharing the way we felt with each other.

We also came to realize that the side effects of some PD medications—beyond the basic stress of an incurable condition—were making our marriage even harder.

In retrospect, much of Gil's compulsiveness was related to the dopamine agonist he was on. He tried two. Both agonists have been ditched.

His unattractive behaviors included impulsive spending (like buying a new car without consulting me or the family budget), increased sexual libido, feelings of self-importance, the need for constant praise, and being overly enthusiastic about whatever his latest endeavor was. His daughter once asked me if he was OK because his recent phone conversations with her were uncharacteristically long and jubilant.

Gil and I now joke together about his being "too close to the end of the diving board" when one of those over-exuberant occasions presents itself, although it happens much less frequently.

Whatever lies down the road with Parkinson's, this care partner is very glad she has a therapist on speed dial.

[See Appendix E: Early Diagnosis Matters because of the painful impact undiagnosed PD has on relationships]

●   ●   ●

Lesson Learned

A social worker/therapist is vital to a care team—for both Parkie and care partner—because the medications and stress of Parkinson's take a tremendous toll on a marriage. Even if one thinks the marriage is solid and open, it's worthwhile having several sessions to be sure no stumbling blocks exist as a couple face "PD life" together.

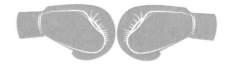

CHAPTER 9:

Care-Partner Abyss

(by Struby Thelen)

Who am I to be writing about care-partner stress? I'm a relative newbie at this.

Many of you have been at it much longer. You *know* about living in the Parkinson's chaos. You've lost jobs, freedom, dreams, well-being, daily rhythms, and the spouse you knew so well. At times, I'm sure you've felt more fear, loneliness, grief, worry, impatience, sadness, exhaustion, and anger than I have yet. I'm learning as I go, trying to prepare for the journey ahead.

I believe God does not give us more than we can handle, and He helps those who help themselves. I have faith He will give me the courage and strength to do what needs to be done when the times come, and faith that I will have done what I can to make the best of Gil's and my life together.

I am a planner. I am most comfortable knowing or setting a goal, exploring the options for reaching it, thus having an idea of likely outcomes. I do a worst-case analysis first (to the great chagrin of my husband), then best-case analysis, and figure the ultimate outcome is somewhere in between. Just knowing I have plans in place for the most probable outcomes gives me a sense of preparedness.

As Gil loves to say, Parkinson's is the worst possible condition for someone like me to manage. He is so right. *Nothing* is certain. *Nothing* is the same hour-to-hour, much less day-to-day. *Nothing* (a mood, an ache, an urge) can be fully explained. The end result is rarely known, and certainly there is no "probable" path.

PD is a condition of rigidity, and I have to become infinitely flexible to deal with it. Gil and I both are learning what situations stress each other and ways to reduce them so our life together will go more smoothly.

For me, that means giving up knowing so many details. Planning for potential outcomes is pretty useless. I have given up trying to keep my surroundings as neat and organized as I'd like, given up thinking I can do it all myself, and focus more on the here and now with my husband.

Go with the flow.

Because so many ups and downs make up a Parkie's day, I have an almost unlimited number of "if-then"s continually to plan for. It is exhausting. This "planning" is the hardest thing for me to let go. I keep telling myself simply to be prepared for whatever happens next. A favorite phrase of ours has become: It all depends.

- I build in more time to prepare myself for an activity, in case Gil needs me to do something for him that I might not be expecting.

- Some PD medications can cause drowsiness. Soon after going on the medication Sinemet, Gil would have to turn the driving over to me when he suddenly got sleepy. I now brace myself to do more of the driving, even though I'd much rather be the passenger/navigator and read, talk, or sew. I also glance at him behind the wheel more often to make sure he's alert and not starting to nod off, as he did once.

- If Gil decides it is less stressful for him to drive the long route home, I take a deep breath and squelch the urge to say it would have been faster to go another way. For him, to keep moving is more important than miles or minutes.

- Gil moves more slowly. His mental speed is slower. His physical movements are slower. He cannot multitask as he used to. I routinely allow him extra time. For example, if he says he'll be home in 2 hours I add an additional 30 to 45 minutes before I actually expect him to pull into the garage or try to check in with him.

- Traveling is more stressful. Where is the closest restroom going to be? Is he likely to get jostled by a crowd? How uneven is the walking surface? How can I efficiently pack all the things we might need? I now try to carry more of his items and oversee both our belongings through air-port security, for example. I occasionally accompany him on business trips just for fun and so I'm there if he needs something, though I will have no role at the destination.

- Gil and I have synced our phone calendars, so each of us knows what the other's schedule is before making our own plans and to remind each other of upcoming events.

- I try not to talk as much about weighty subjects when Gil is driving, so he can concentrate on where he is going and the traffic around us. I try to plan my need for details around what he is doing or how he is feeling at the time.

- Gil was worried one day because he was going to have to fill out a bunch of papers and I was not going to be there to write his answers. I suggested he matter-of-factly tell the person that he had Parkinson's, and they would have to do the writing since his handwriting was no longer legible. It must have gone better than expected, because he has used similar lines often since then, and others have responded calmly and respectfully.

- I enjoy knowing details because they give me specific information I can use to plan, make decisions, whatever. But fine points are often lost or forgotten by someone with Parkinson's. I am learning to operate with less information and to be more forgiving when things are forgotten, and Gil is learning to put up with my need for minutiae and my reminders.

Live with more clutter.

Neat surroundings calm me. Clutter is stressful.

- I try to give Gil the space to do as much for himself as he can. In Tampa, he had taken over a bathroom that I thought needed to be clean in case company dropped by. His backup bathroom became a little-used one. I rarely went into it, so I didn't have to look at the clutter that would drive me crazy or worry about unexpected guests seeing the mess.

- We've added more Parkinson's "stuff" in our household. Weighted tableware now nestles beside the forks and spoons in the cutlery drawer. I've trashed little-used glass-ware to make room for his handled glasses and mugs, which are easier to hold.

- Cigar smokers deal with a lot of natural clutter: home humidor, multiple traveling humidors, cigar cutters, an array of lighters, butane cans to refill empty lighters, cigars, cigar wrappers, cigar bands, ashtrays, ashes and more ashes. Gil tries to keep his porch "office" neat, but many of those items he used to keep tucked away are now in plain view. Putting them away promptly would mean him taking many more steps around the house. I try not to make him feel obligated to get up and down from a chair any more than he feels like it at any given moment.

- Instead of trying to keep "public" areas of the house constantly neat, I do a sweeping pick-up just before company arrives. Unexpected drop-ins will just have to understand that the foot-stool or small table is there to assist Gil, even though it does not fit with the decor.

- Clothes don't get picked up or hung up as often as they did. So be it.

I am not Superwoman.

Multi-tasking used to be a specialty of mine. I easily juggled being a newspaper editor's wife, middle school PTSA officer, elementary school PTA president, school newsletter editor, Cub Scout den leader, assistant Boy Scout leader, and a member of multiple tennis teams. I expected perfection from myself in every role. These days, my outside responsibilities are significantly reduced so I have more time for Gil.

- Nurturing the "us" in our marriage is important to the journey. I continue to evaluate things on my to-do list and tackle those that I think are most meaningful to our marriage, and hand off or ignore the less important ones. Spending time with him, for example, is more important to me than keeping the house as clean as I once did. Downsizing with our Macon home has helped considerably.

- I still need to vocalize my stresses earlier so Gil better understands why I sometimes respond the way I do.

I have always had a good sense of direction, but on a visit to Bethesda, MD, Gil got out of the car at the restaurant entrance so he would not have to walk so far, and I drove in search of a parking spot. I had never driven in that area and finally found a parking garage seemingly some five or six blocks away, on a side street of a side street. I got turned around walking back to the restaurant. Frustrated, I called Gil for the address, but he did not answer because he'd left his phone in the car. After finding the address online on my phone, I got to the table about 30 minutes later.

The next day Gil asked if I would drop him at the airport curb with our bags, return our rental car, and take the shuttle back to the airport. I said since he was used to driving around that airport, I'd manage the bags instead.

The following day, I could tell Gil was annoyed about something. When he said he was frustrated because I had him return the rental car, I burst into tears. I had been so stressed about uncharacteristically getting lost walking to the restaurant the day before that all I could think about was: What if I get lost trying to find the rental car return and we miss the flight home? If I'd explained why I wanted *him* to return the rental car instead of *me*, I suspect he would have avoided being piqued.

- Support networks are important. While I am not comfortable—at least right now—in joining a care-partner therapy group, I am very thankful for PD support groups where ideas, answers, and resources can be exchanged among Parkies and care partners, and for private therapy to help with specific issues.

- Gil was always the big-picture partner in our marriage. I figured out the details and carried out the plan. Together we are assembling a group of advisors (financial, tax, legal, for example) who I know I can rely on when the time comes.

- Down the road, I am prepared to ask others to help me help Gil. We were pro-active in exploring options for down-sizing that resulted in being closer to family and a terrific place that offers graduated steps of assisted living.

Together is better.

Gil's and my journeys always will be different, but we no longer shut each other out. Parkinson's does not define our "new normal" life together, although it significantly shapes it.

- Gil has gotten to know more of my friends and introduced me to more of his. I am blessed to have new good friends just because our paths crossed through Parkinson's. Gil even attended a Dinner Done monthly meals-prep session I did with Tampa friends for more than 12 years to see first-hand what it was all about.

- His energy levels vary, and we can't do some things we used to enjoy doing together. That Tampa Parkinson's spinning class at the Y would improve my health as well as his, so I went with him when my tennis permitted.

- We have significantly more common goals these days and are much more respectful of the activities that are meaningful in each other's lives. Gil still immerses himself in his community and PD work, and I am included in activities important to him, like writing this book. He understands tennis is a large part of my social and exercise life and will attend a match occasionally to cheer my team on.

Early on I was asked what it felt like to be a care partner. I didn't know because in those days I didn't feel like a care partner. I didn't feel included enough in his life to understand what he was going through, and ways to help him were fairly straight-forward.

PD has progressed. We are talking more candidly, and I have a much greater sense of what he needs and expects from me. I am confident he has a better understanding of what I need and expect from him. That knowledge, thanks to our therapist, has helped relieve a significant amount of stress for both of us.

After a Parkinson's support group meeting at which Gil spoke, a woman came to me with tears in her eyes. In a cracking voice she asked, "What can I do to help my husband?" I responded: "Ask him what he'd like for you to do."

Parkies struggle to maintain their independence and not be a burden to their loved ones. For care partners (and family and friends), assuming and doing too much can rob what independence is still there, and doing too little can make your partner feel like he has to beg for help.

I've found that asking if Gil would like for me to help with his socks, for example, gives him the freedom to say "no"—when he's having a good day and can do it himself—or "yes"—if he's having a bad Parkie day.

● ● ●

Lesson Learned

Care partners need to understand their own as well as their Parkie's stress points and find ways to reduce them, while being respectful of what their partner's limits are at any given time.

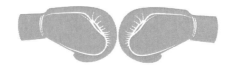

CHAPTER 10:

The Magic of PD SELF

Diane Cook is a wisp of a woman, whom I lovingly call Brain. She's changed my life.

I met Diane and her husband Gary in 2016. They led the training of teams who would lead PD SELF programs in nine test sites, including Tampa.

Diane, a Parkie herself, explained the program this way on her PD SELF website:

"Many people are handed a diagnosis with very little guidance on what to do next. But the diagnosis is life changing. Facing life with a chronic progressive disease means facing changes to health, relationships, family life, employment and finances.

"Research tells us that when people are given the resources to cope with these changes, they are empowered to take an active role in managing PD, leading to better health and quality of life.

"PD Self-Efficacy Learning Forum (PD SELF) is an innovative disease management program that offers this approach. ...

"Based on the psychosocial theory of self-efficacy, PD SELF helps people newly diagnosed with PD to create a personalized approach to managing their disease. Self-efficacy is the confidence

a person has in his or her ability to influence an outcome or be successful in achieving a result. Self-efficacy beliefs determine how people think, feel and motivate themselves. It is increasingly used in health care for its effectiveness in helping people to adopt healthier behaviors.

"A central focus of PD SELF is to help people strengthen self-efficacy beliefs, thereby positively influencing the management of their disease. At the end of the first clinical trial testing this approach, researchers found that PD SELF:

- *Improved mental health and well-being of people with PD and their care partners.*

- *Decreased participants' stress, anxiety and depression, and improved sleep.*

- *Improved participants' emotional well-being, even when PD (or general health) declined.*

- *Led to long-term improvement in the areas above, with changes observed for as long as four years after the clinical trial ended.*

- *Led participants to become more active in the Parkinson's community, for example through increased enrollment in clinical trials."*

That's PD SELF in a nutshell.

In my terms, it's a "vertical" assault against PD. It fits my aggressive temperament and beliefs perfectly. I added its practices and tools to my arsenal of counterpunches.

In action in Tampa for me, PD SELF was 34 Parkies and care partners meeting for nine monthly, 2½-hour sessions in a renovated downtown church. Each session included expert presentations on key information: exercise, diet, non-motor symptoms, drugs, causation, far-reaching discussions, and exercises to build mental power.

Building and managing a personal health-care team is the paramount goal of the training. Each person's team will be different.

[See Appendix F: Your Health-Care Team]

The backbone of my team includes University of Florida Movement Disorder Specialist (MDS) neurologist Adolfo Ramirez-Zamora (an associate of the remarkable neurologist Michael Okun) and Macon gerontologist Jayesh Patel.

I am team captain. I expect to add other specialists, such as an occupational therapist and a speech therapist, as the condition progresses.

An unusual support group was born in Tampa among PD SELF participants. Not surprisingly, its leaders were people already in Rock Steady Boxing programs. They were early adopters of the **vertical** message.

The camaraderie and sociability of support groups have appreciable health benefits, which physicians ignore at their peril.

A compelling book, *A General Theory of Love*, explains the neurophysiological reason that properly structured support groups—such as PD SELF—are so vital for overcoming health challenges.

".... One study, for instance, found that social isolation tripled the death rate following a heart attack. Another found that going to group psychotherapy doubled the postsurgical lifespan of women with breast cancer. A third noted that leukemia patients with strong social supports had two-year survival rates more than twice that of those who lacked them.

"In his fascinating book 'Love & Survival', Dean Ornish surveyed the medical literature on the relationship between isolation and human mortality. His conclusion: dozens of studies demonstrate that solitary people have a vastly increased rate of premature death from all causes—they are three to five times likelier to die earlier than people with ties to a caring spouse, family or community.

"With results like these backing the medical efficacy of mammalian congregation, you might think that treatments like group therapy after breast cancer would be standard.

"Guess again. Affiliation is not a drug or an operation, and that makes it nearly invisible to Western medicine. Our doctors are not uninformed; on the contrary, most have read these studies and grant them a grudging intellectual acceptance.

"But they don't **believe** (book authors' emphasis) in them; they can't bring themselves to base treatment decisions on a rumored phantom like attachment. The prevailing medical paradigm has no capacity to incorporate the concept that a relationship is a physiologic process, as real and as potent as any pill or surgical procedure."

The Parkinson's Alliance, a patient advocacy group, reported in 2017 more evidence that social support is vital for Parkies.

"Data was gathered from 1,421 individuals with PD. Many participants said they have strong support systems, inclusive of family, friends, significant others, the medical community, and the PD community.

"Despite strong support systems, PD increased strain on family and care providers for 40% of participants. Forty-nine percent reported moderately to extremely reduced access to support, resulting in changed relationships.

"Symptoms adversely impacted the quality of support from others for 77% of participants. Fatigue, motor symptoms, speech disturbance and cognitive and emotional disturbance were the most highly reported barriers to a strong support system."

Writing in The New York Times in 2016, Dr. Dhruv Khulllar of Harvard Medical School, said:

"Social isolation is a growing epidemic—one that's increasingly recognized as having dire physical, mental and emotional consequences. Since the 1980s, the percentage of American adults who say they're lonely has doubled from 20 percent to 40 percent.

"About one-third of Americans older than 65 now live alone, and half of those over 85 do. People in poorer health—especially those with mood disorders like anxiety and depression—are more likely to feel lonely. Those without a college education are the least likely to have someone they can talk to about important personal matters.

"A wave of new research suggests social separation is bad for us. Individuals with less social connection have disrupted sleep patterns, altered immune systems, more inflammation and higher levels of stress hormones. One recent study found that isolation increases the risk of heart disease by 29 percent and stroke by 32 percent.

"Another analysis that pooled data from 70 studies and 3.4 million people found that socially isolated individuals had a 30 percent higher risk of dying in the next seven years, and that this effect was largest in middle age.

"Loneliness can accelerate cognitive decline in older adults, and isolated individuals are twice as likely to die prematurely as those with more robust social interactions. These effects start early: Socially isolated children have significantly poorer health 20 years later, even after controlling for other factors. All told, loneliness is as important a risk factor for early death as obesity and smoking.

"The evidence on social isolation is clear. What to do about it is less so.

"Loneliness is an especially tricky problem because accepting and declaring our loneliness carries profound stigma. Admitting we're lonely can feel as if we're admitting we've failed in life's most fundamental domains: belonging, love, attachment. It attacks our basic instincts to save face, and makes it hard to ask for help."

Sociability case closed.

•   •   •

Lessons Learned

Combine extensive research and mental confidence to build your health-care team.

A broad and deep social network aids your well-being.

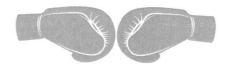

CHAPTER 11:

A Better Road

We all die. My question is: "Under what circumstances?"

Like Tom Graboys, I want my last days to be joyous, surrounded by people who matter to me, people I love. Let there be laughter, storytelling, music, and wine.

I will raise my glass to toast the words of Mario de Andrade in *"The Valuable Time of Maturity"*:

"My goal is to reach the end satisfied and at peace with my loved ones and my conscience."

I want my friend and collaborator Kirk Hall with me at the joyful end.

Kirk is a bear of a man. That, and his rumbling voice, command attention. He's usually the smartest guy in the room, and people know it. I do.

Kirk was and is a marketer. His product now is a cause: better lives for fellow Parkies. He blogs and writes books about PD, his best known being *"Window of Opportunity."*

We met electronically in 2015. Each of us was urging the then-Parkinson Disease Foundation (PDF) to make palliative care that year's topic of concern. PDF did. We each wrote proposals.

Kirk and I were together for the first time in Denver in October 2015 for an international meeting of healthcare professionals, PD patients, and their care partners. The subject was reshaping palliative care specifically for Parkinson's.

The council of Parkies and care partners urged far-reaching changes in PD care. Kirk and I were principal authors of the final report published in the online journal *Nature* in 2017. In it, we invoke the memory of Tom Graboys and his clinical greatness. Excerpts from our report follow:

"… The council endorses palliative care as an approach to the care of Parkinson's disease patients and their families that seeks to reduce suffering through spiritual, psychosocial, and medical support. This approach should start at the time of diagnosis, as this is a very challenging time for patients and care partners; includes better emotional support, educational resources, and closer follow-up than is currently standard; and continues through end-of-life care and bereavement.

"… The Graboys allegory contains many of the early stage recommendations of our own prescription for PD Palliative Care and is based on the approach Graboys took with his own patients. While such an approach may not fit every physician or patient, we hope it provides some useful examples of patient-centered care for PD. …

"We envision a new, improved approach to Palliative Care based on a 'three-legged stool' including the patient's primary care physician and neurologist (leg 1), a PD palliative care team (leg 2), and a PD support entity (leg 3). The 'three legs' are meant to provide support for patients, care partners, and families throughout the PD journey.

"Early Stage: Diagnosis to 5 Years (Honeymoon Period)

"Given confusion and misperceptions about palliative care, we suggest using the term 'supportive care' and discussing this

concept as PD Life Enhancement, or something similar. Palliative care should provide a comprehensive, coordinated, and consistent approach for the medical and PD support communities designed to maximize quality of life for patients, care partners, and families starting at diagnosis and to reduce stress for the duration of the disease and bereavement period.

"The key points for diagnosis were included in the Graboys allegory. Another important element is sharing informational resources. ... We recommend scheduling follow-up a month after diagnosis since many patients are 'shell-shocked' and unable to absorb much beyond the words PD. This is an opportunity for the doctor to assess how the patient and care partner are doing, ask if they have reviewed information resources, and answer questions....

"We recommend an appointment a year after diagnosis to assess the patient's and care partner's 'readiness' to be provided with additional informational resources. ... Most people should be ready at that point and some may have already begun this process on their own. If not, we recommend discussing why they are not ready.

"Some patients take the 'what I don't know won't hurt me' approach. It is important to share that in general, patients and care partners who do best in managing PD take 'ownership' of it so that they can properly advocate for themselves and make good choices.

"We recommend participation in self-efficacy or chronic disease management education programs. This is also a good time to revisit the potential benefits of joining a support group. The doctor should have a working relationship with regional and local support groups. ...

"Middle Stage: 5 Years to Advent of Symptoms that Substantially Affect Daily Living

"The middle stage is a crucial time for patients, care partners, and families. It is a time when learning can take place relative to late stage. Plans and decisions can be made to make the later stage easier. Wrestling with these issues, including faith, can create acceptance and peace of mind, making the last stage of the journey far less stressful.

"Tasks should include:

- Prepare a personal plan for taking ownership of possible outcomes, including the possibility of financial challenges.

- Develop end-of-life wish list and legal documents including advance directives.

- Discuss with doctor what his/her role will be in end stage.

- Discuss care partner plan for assistance and self-care.

- Begin assessing need for in-home safety and for equipment.

- Consider counseling to address faith/spiritual issues or concerns.

"Many patients, care partners, and families miss this extremely important opportunity for a variety of reasons. They may not have as much warning as they think before they are in the thick of late stage and end up scurrying around to find resources, fighting among themselves at a time when they need to be focused on caring for each other. They may not want to face the inevitable decline of their loved one and the difficult decisions this entails, so they take the 'ostrich' approach by sticking their heads in the sand. PD palliative care clinics may have value in helping families in this stage.

"Late Stage: Advent of Significant Disability/ Hospice to Death/Bereavement

"In our model, the late stage becomes a matter of implementing plans and preferences identified in the middle stage including hospice when appropriate. Legal paperwork will be available to minimize confusion, misunderstandings, or other 'bumps in the road.' Of course, it is not likely that all developments can be foreseen and planned for, but these should be the exception. If the plan includes contingencies based on the nature of specific health issues as they unfold, there can be 'course adjustments' as opposed to confusion and stress related to confrontation of unanticipated issues.

"… From our perspective it seems that many neurologists are uncomfortable remaining involved after they can no longer 'fix' their patient. Training in palliative care or involvement of palliative medicine specialists could help remedy this issue.

"It is extremely important to be mindful of care partner stress/ burnout at this stage, and this is an area where a palliative care team could and should add great value. The team needs to be aware that the care partner can become so overwhelmed that they do not take the time or have the energy to reach out for help. …

"Medical Community Proposal

"We proposed a fundamental shift in the mindset and training of doctors starting in medical school to facilitate the changes discussed, including getting to know patients and care partners beyond their medical records and the importance of remaining engaged in late stage to help ensure a 'successful transition to death.' We would describe this as one in which the care partner, family, and medical team can feel at peace because they did everything possible to honor the patient's wishes about how he/ she wanted to die.

"… Another recommended area of focus for medical schools is the ethical aspects of working with patients who would be better served elsewhere. This is a sensitive subject because it shines a spotlight on doctors who choose to continue treating a patient despite knowing better options exist. We have seen many patients in our support groups receive inappropriate treatments or be *incorrectly told there is nothing more to offer by doctors without PD-specific knowledge or skills."*

This, I believe, is A Better Road for the Parkinson's journey. I hope you do, too.

[See Appendix G: the full article of Palliative Care for Parkinson's Disease and its two resources lists]

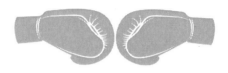

CHAPTER 12.

Making "Good Trouble"

Parkinson's is a Monster: Infinite symptoms. Multiple causes. No treatment template.

If cancer is the "Emperor of Diseases," Parkinson's is the "Enigma of (Neurological) Conditions."

Parkinson's complexity in diagnosing and treating is a trapdoor for sufferers, inviting passivity and inertia. Life on the couch. The horizontal default option.

The vertical option—fighting back—requires commitment and perseverance.

Fighting back starts with valid, actionable information. With that, empowerment is possible,

I acquired both in PD SELF training. (Chapter 10)

Eight PD SELF grads and their care partners in Tampa formed an unusual support group, the Parkinson's Disease Action Group (PDAG). I described it this way in our Mission Statement:

"No accountability organization or system exists for strongly aspirational and persevering Parkies. We have created one.

"Our goal is to help one another out-wit, out-flank, and counterpunch this unwelcome tenant in our brains.

"We will share and learn from one another's action steps, such as second-and-more opinions, off-label medications, busting through bureaucratic barriers, and workarounds for diminished skills and loss of control.

"We will persevere. Promise made. Promise to be delivered."

PDAG's action program is development of a groundbreaking program—Me-Over-PD (MOPD)—to reach newly diagnosed people with Parkinson's. Those newly diagnosed individuals will receive—for the first time anywhere—real-time, verified, actionable, local information to assist them in navigating this mysterious condition.

The consortium comprises the PDAG group and several faculty members of the University of South Florida's Zimmerman School of Advertising & Mass Communications.

The heart of MOPD is a live database of crucial resources, including neurologists specializing in mobility diseases, physical therapists, speech therapists, occupational therapists, dietitians, and personal trainers, to name a few.

No such database exists anywhere for the newly diagnosed Parkinson's person and his/her general practitioner or treating neurologist. Existing "help lines" have limited, highly local information and lack resources for constant verification and updating.

The database will be used to prepare a brochure ("Road Map") distributed through hospitals, neurology clinics, drug stores, YMCAs, agencies for the aging, and doctors' offices, to name several.

The target audience, for starters, is Parkinson's sufferers in the northern Tampa Bay region. Based upon lessons learned from the northern Tampa Bay rollout, MOPD intends to extend its Tampa Bay reach by partnering with local and regional community support agencies.

We believe that newly diagnosed Parkinson's sufferers can substantially increase the suitability of their treatments along with the quality of their lives if they are fully informed of what resources are needed, where these resources are available, and how to access them.

MOPD is a Florida non-profit corporation. It received 501(c)(3) approval in April 2018.

MOPD plans to be operational by the end of 2019. Janelle Applequist, assistant professor at the Zimmerman School is leading operations. I am president.

I work in two geographic and Parkie communities. One is the northern Tampa Bay region (Hillsborough, Pinellas, and Pasco counties) where Struby and I lived happily for almost 20 years.

The second is Macon, GA, where Struby and I moved in November 2017. Our new home is the splendid continuing-care community, Carlyle Place.

We moved to be closer to family.

Struby is from Macon. Her brother Neil Struby and sister-in-law Hazel live there, and niece Hazel Caldwell's family is in nearby Forsyth.

My brother Neil Thelen, his wife Norma, my nephew Mark's family and Struby's nephew Neil's family are all about two hours away in the Atlanta suburbs.

Struby has potential help should my Parkinson's progression go badly, such as severe dementia. I preach preparedness. I need to live it.

In Macon, Struby and I host meetings for Parkies and care partners to discuss the nuances of PD and design action steps to improve care for all patients in Middle Georgia. We call those "Study/Action Groups."

Typically, each group meets six times, over two months, with each session running about 90 minutes. Our group size has been roughly seven Parkies, plus their care partners.

Participants are asked to read and absorb chapters in "Counterpunch" prior to each session. I do not "teach" in the formal sense. I lead discussions of the topic. The focus is what group members will *do* with the information to live well, or at least better, with their PD.

We also use the Parkinson's Foundation superb *Q&A* and the DPF's comprehensive *Every Victory Counts (EVC)*. (As mentioned earlier, you can order or download both free. The *Q&A* at <u>www.parkinson.org/pd-library/books/Q-and-A-Seventh-Edition</u> and the *EVC* at <u>www.davisphinneyfoundation.org/resources/every-victory-counts-2017/</u>.)

The "syllabus" we used in 2018 was this:

Session 1/Introduction: What we will do; roles and responsibilities

Session 2/Discovering What PD Is: Causes; symptoms

Session 3/Fighting Back: Exercise, exercise, exercise, exercise; diet; mental toughness; camaraderie; health-care team; workarounds; neuroplasticity

Session 4/Inner Living with PD: What it is like; how you are perceived by family, friends, and others

Session 5/Care Partner Stress

Session 6/Structural Reform: Me Over PD; palliative care retooling

In addition to the Study/Action Groups, I am working with Mercer University's medical school to improve Parkinson's awareness among current and future physicians.

As of mid-2018, Georgia lacks a care system for patients to enter for guidance and assistance in making necessary lifestyle improvements. Those include diet, exercise, social engagement, and mental discipline.

Struby and I are a working to pool the assets of Middle Georgia university and health-care organizations to create a patient-driven "system" of care. That is our "Good Trouble-Making."

Struby has assembled a list of local resources recommended by patients and care partners to assist Parkies in carrying out their individual wellness plans. We refer to it as "MOPD Lite."

Doing both the system and MOPD Lite, we believe, will move Georgia to the front rank of states doing well by citizens who are fighting back against their enigmatic malady.

Struby and I wish you the best in "Living Well With Parkinson's."

GLOSSARY

Alpha-synuclein: A protein in Lewy bodies, clumps that are the pathological hallmark of Parkinson's.

Bradykinesia: Slowed movement and impaired ability to move swiftly on command. It's most commonly a symptom of Parkinson's and a main thing doctors look for when diagnosing Parkinson's.

Bradyphrenia: Slowness of thought, common to many disorders of the brain.

Carbidopa-levodopa: Also known as levocarb and co-carbidopa, is the combination of the two medications carbidopa and levodopa. It is prescribed to manage Parkinson's symptoms. Sinemet is one brand name.

Dopamine: In non-technical terms, dopamine is the "WD-40" brain chemical that facilitates communication between nerves and muscles.

Dyskinesia: Involuntary muscle movements and diminished voluntary movements. Dyskinesia ranges from a slight hand tremor to uncontrollable movement of the upper body or lower extremities.

Dystonia: Repetitive muscle contractions that result in twisting and repetitive movements or abnormal fixed postures.

Forced exercise: Exercise intensity greater than accustomed, such as sprinting on a bicycle rather than cruising.

Lewy body: An abnormal deposit of the protein alpha-synuclein in the brain. Those deposits can diminish thinking, movement, behavior, and mood.

Lewy body dementia: Sometimes called Lewy body disorder, includes Parkinson's dementia and dementia with Lewy bodies—two dementias characterized by super-abnormal deposits of alpha-synuclein in the brain.

MDS: Movement Disorder Specialist, a neurologist with two additional years of training in neuromuscular disorders, such as Parkinson's and Huntington's.

Neurogenesis: The process by which neurons are produced by neural stem cells. It is most active during embryonic development but occurs throughout life.

Neuroplasticity: The ability of the brain to change throughout life. Brain activity of a function, for example mechanics of a golf swing, can be transferred to a different brain location after injury.

Neurorestoration: Restoration of a brain function through new neurons or new neural pathways.

Palliative care: A multidisciplinary approach to specialized medical and nursing care for people with life-limiting illnesses. It provides relief from the symptoms, pain, and stress of a terminal diagnosis.

PWP or Parkie, Parkies: Person or people with Parkinson's.

Sinemet: The brand name of the combination medicine that contains the drugs levodopa and carbidopa.

Visuospatial impairment: The process of the brain accurately locating objects in space. It determines how far objects are from you and from each other. Visuospatial impairments or deficits link to driving problems (lane drifting, hitting curbs, crooked parking) and misjudging bodily distances (bumping into corners of tables, knocking over drinking glasses).

Bodily Symptoms Checklist

Building on Dr. David E. Riley's classification of Parkinson's symptoms, Parkies can expect to experience some of the following. Which are you experiencing?

Motor Symptoms:

- ☐ Drooling, swallowing problems
- ☐ Weak voice
- ☐ Facial masking
- ☐ Difficulty turning over in bed
- ☐ Rigidity, painful stiffness
- ☐ Hand/leg tremors
- ☐ Hesitation, freezing in place
- ☐ Loss of dexterity, fine motor skills, including a change in handwriting
- ☐ Muscle spasms, cramps
- ☐ Restless legs syndrome
- ☐ Decrease in natural arm swing
- ☐ Shuffling gait, smaller steps
- ☐ Twisting posture*
- ☐ Walking problems, difficulty turning the body

☐ Stooped/unstable posture

☐ Slowed movements

Non-Motor Symptoms:

Cognitive:

☐ Articulation, slurred speech

☐ Reduced executive function

☐ Communication

☐ Attention, working memory

☐ Decision-making

☐ Difficulty finding the "right" word

☐ Memory

☐ Slower processing skills, slow thinking

☐ Weak voice

☐ Visuospatial issues

Psychiatric:

☐ Anxiety

☐ Confusion

☐ Impulse control disorders (gambling, spending, sex, energy, eating)*

☐ Depression, sadness

☐ Apathy

☐ Euphoria

☐ Fatigue, loss of energy*

☐ Hallucinations* (hearing, touching, smelling, seeing, or tasting something that isn't there)

☐ Delusions, illusions* (a belief, for example, that someone is trying to poison them or is stealing one's belongings)

- ☐ Mood swings*
- ☐ Loss of pleasure

Autonomic Nervous System:

- ☐ Blood pressure regulation
- ☐ Breathing difficulties
- ☐ Constipation/diarrhea
- ☐ Fainting, lightheadedness, dizziness*
- ☐ Too little sweating
- ☐ Bladder control
- ☐ Frequent nighttime urination
- ☐ Dry/oily face/scalp
- ☐ Nausea*
- ☐ Weight loss/gain*
- ☐ Balance, equilibrium issues
- ☐ Hot/cold flashes
- ☐ Dry eyes, decreased blinking
- ☐ Rash, skin redness
- ☐ Mole changes
- ☐ Increased risk of melanoma skin cancer
- ☐ Impotence, loss of orgasm
- ☐ Increased/decreased libido*
- ☐ Swelling of ankles/legs

Sensory:

- ☐ Loss of smell
- ☐ Change in vision acuity
- ☐ Double vision*
- ☐ Blurry vision*
- ☐ Itching
- ☐ Numbness, tingling, loss of feeling in hands/fingers
- ☐ Color vision issues

Sleep:

- ☐ Insomnia
- ☐ Sleep apnea, breathing pauses
- ☐ Excessive daytime sleepiness*
- ☐ Talking/yelling while asleep
- ☐ REM sleep disorder (acting out vivid, violent, and vocal nightmares)
- ☐ Change in sleep patterns
- ☐ Difficulty staying asleep
- ☐ Open eyes while asleep

* Some of these issues also could be treatment-related side effects.

[Expanded from Davis Phinney Foundation for Parkinson's Body Symptom Map, Parkinson Foundation website, American Parkinson Disease Association website, "Common PD Symptoms and Treatment Side Effects" from the University at Buffalo Neurology, and personal experience.]

The rogue protein behind Parkinson's disease may also protect your gut

By Meredith Wadman
Science Magazine

The hallmark brain damage in Parkinson's disease is thought to be the work of a misfolded, rogue protein **that spreads from brain cell to brain cell like an infection**. Now, researchers have found that the normal form of the protein—α-synuclein (αS)—may actually defend the intestines against invaders by marshaling key immune cells. But chronic intestinal infections could ultimately cause Parkinson's, the scientists suggest, if αS migrates from over-loaded nerves in the gut wall to the brain.

"The gut-brain immune axis seems to be on a cusp of an explosion of new insights, and this work offers an exceptionally exciting new hypothesis," says Charles Bevins, an expert in intestinal immunity at the University of California, Davis, who was not involved with the study.

The normal function of αS has long been a mystery. Though the protein is known to accumulate in toxic clumps in the brain and the nerves of the gut wall in patients with Parkinson's disease, no one was sure what it did in healthy people. Noting that a region of the αS molecule behaves similarly to small, microbe-targeting proteins that are part of the body's immune defenses, Michael Zasloff, an immunologist at Georgetown University Medical Center in Washington, D.C., set out to find whether aS, too, might help fend off microbial invaders.

To see whether aS was indeed playing a role in the gut's immune defenses, Zasloff, Ethan Stolzenberg of the University of Oklahoma Health Sciences Center in Oklahoma City, and their colleagues spent 9 years collecting and analyzing biopsies of the duodenum—the first part of the intestine where nerves normally produce very little aS—from 42 children unlikely to have Parkinson's disease. (The early stages of the disease virtually never appear until adulthood.) The children had abdominal pain, diarrhea, vomiting, and other gastrointestinal symptoms, along with gut inflammation visible under a microscope. The scientists found that the aS protein was indeed present in the nerves of the inflamed intestine—and the more intensely inflamed the tissue was, the more aS the team found.

But was the aS a cause or an effect of the inflammation? To find out, the researchers turned to biopsies from 14 children and two adults who received intestinal transplants and later developed infections with norovirus, a common gut pathogen. In most, the aS protein was abundantly evident during infection. In four of nine patients—whose intestines had been biopsied before, during, and after the infection—the aS protein appeared only during the infection, but not before. (Zasloff conjectures that the five patients who showed aS production prior to infection were making it in response to another, pre-existing viral infection.)

Next, the scientists asked whether the aS protein was acting as a magnet for inflammatory cells, which are a key part of a normal immune response. In lab dish experiments, they found that aS, whether in its normal conformation or in the misfolded aggregates found in Parkinson's disease, powerfully attracted white blood cells that are present in both acute and chronic inflammation. They also discovered that both forms of aS activated dendritic cells, which lead to lasting immunity by presenting bits of foreign invaders to lymphocytes—the white blood cells that "remember" specific microbial intruders and respond in force to later invasions. After exposing immature dendritic cells to αS for 48 hours, the team discovered that the more αS, the more dendritic cells were activated. Together, **the data suggest the production of** αS **by nerves in the gut wall is the cause—and not the effect—of tissue inflammation**, the authors write today in the *Journal of Innate Immunity*. "This discovery shows us that the [gut's] nervous system can play a key role in both health and disease," Zasloff says.

The authors note that people with multiple copies of the gene that directs the production of αS inevitably develop Parkinson's disease—in essence, production of the protein overwhelms the body's ability to clear it, and it forms the toxic aggregates that cause Parkinson's. They also write that repeated acute or chronic gut infections could produce "a comparable increase" in αS.

The paper's findings are "thrilling," says Aletta Kraneveld, an immunopharmacologist who studies the gut-brain axis at the University of Utrecht in the Netherlands. "This is the first [study] showing that a protein very, very relevant for Parkinson's disease is able to induce an immune response. It opens up so many avenues for new research."

Zasloff himself is moving into the clinic, treating Parkinson's patients for constipation using a synthetic version of squalamine, a natural steroid made by the dogfish shark. Squalamine, says Zasloff, prompts bowel movement and blocks αS action in gut wall nerves. The early phase trial is being conducted by Enterin, a Philadelphia, Pennsylvania–based firm Zasloff founded with his co-author, neurologist Denise Barbut, now Enterin's chief medical officer. If the drug succeeds in reversing constipation, the researchers will conclude that it has disrupted the function of αS in the intestinal nerves. "This type of approach could also in principle alter the whole natural history of the disease," Zasloff says.

But David Beckham, a neurovirologist and physician at the University of Denver, is cautious. "Potentially αS is playing some role in helping neurons fight off infections," he says. But he adds that the current study doesn't do enough to show that it is a cause and not an effect of inflammation.

"This is an early part of a new emerging understanding of what this molecule potentially does," Beckham says. "And I think it's eventually going to lead us in the correct direction as to what's going wrong in Parkinson's disease—and potentially to how can we prevent it."

Bow Ties Pummel Parkinson's

By Gil Thelen
www.ShufflingEditor.com

Cometh a long story about a short tie with large meaning.

I had favored bow ties for 50 years, since graduate school at Cornell Med in New York City.

My collection at peak numbered 37—Foulards, Quads, Links, Felts Pine, Paisley, Lorraine Stripes, Harrisburg Medallions, Snead Neats, Quicksilver Stripes, Becker Stripes, Brooks Stripes, Halstead Spots.

Roll those wonderful names off your tongue.

My bow ties had stories to tell.

I often wondered whether the late Stewart Bryan hired me for Tampa because we both favored short ties. He tied his floppy, telegraphing casual elegance, Virginia-aristocrat branch. (My favorite Bryan quip: "If I had known how rich I was, I would have been drinking better Bourbon all these years.")

Bow tying ended abruptly for me due to Parkinson's. My numb fingers could no longer tie a tie. My now-unused collection stared back at me, kind of angry.

Enter Randy and Veronica.

Randy is the founder of R. Hanauer Bow Ties in Fort Mill, SC, a Charlotte exurb. He made my bow ties for years.

Veronica is the skilled seamstress at the Jos. A. Bank men's clothing store in The Shops at Wiregrass, Wesley Chapel, FL, a Tampa exurb.

A pop-up ad appeared on my computer screen in August. It was for a *pre-tied* bow tie, not an ugly clip-on.

FLASH!

I called Randy. "Do you by chance sell pre-ties?"

"Yes," he answered.

"Can I buy several and would you convert my Hanauer collection to pre-ties?"

Certainly, he said. "Box them up and send them."

Charge?

"None."

Wow!

What about the Brooks Brothers and Ben Silver bow ties I have? Could those be converted?

I showed Veronica the Hanauer pre-ties.

"Can you do the same for my 11 Brooks and Silver ties?"

"I'll try," she answered.

Yesterday I picked the 11 up.

Beautiful work, Veronica. I now have 20 very usable bow ties.

Add an "ankle-biter" to my list of small ways to strike back at Parkinson's, the disease that diminishes a person's powers and saps control of their life.

Gotcha this time, Bruiser!

The Tampa Humidor Trumps My Parkinson's

By Gil Thelen
www.ShufflingEditor.com

It's a 5,000 square-foot storefront hard by railroad tracks in a challenged part of North Tampa. Busch Gardens is two miles east along Busch Boulevard. I-275 is a short mile west.

A Cigar Store Indian silently greets you at the front door. You walk in to the rich aroma of cigars.

The staff is welcoming and endlessly accommodating. Coffee perhaps? A cigar recommendation within your budget? Guidance on accessories from humidors, travel cases to butane lighters and cigar cutters?

Done.

The semi-circular bar faces two 45-inch TVs, always on to sports or news. An oddly misspelled cigar maker's yellow electric sign beckons. "Oliva Serie (cq) V bar."

The bar comfortably seats nine. The Humidor's gracious baristas are busy behind the counter, offering soft drinks, coffee, water, beer, and wine—but no liquor.

The feel is comfortable and welcoming. Quiet readers occupy the 18 stuffed leather chairs and sofa.

The rectangular, 4x10 foot work table seats 8 laptop computer users. They work mostly quietly, sometimes not. (That's chatty me, sometimes.)

One of the six roundtables, with high chairs, is often the "Cribbage Place." Cribbage is the Humidor's signature card game, sometimes raucous, always spirited.

The Humidor opens at 9:30 AM for the coffee regulars (that's you Golf and Cigar Connoisseur Robert) having their initial cigar of the day.

Activity grows around noon. Lunch breakers enjoy a "stick" after their sandwich, (Pre-made Cubans are always available from the back fridge.)

Cribbage players are a backbone of the afternoon crowd. The evening gang is quite different, many of them young professionals.

The Humidor is a male hangout in tone and culture during the day. The occasional female visitor can expect full attention, respectfully. Pepsi Ron, often there, with wife Lorraine says, couples are comfortable because regulars sanitize profane language to fit the mixed-gender setting.

The never-ending parade of buyers, some staying, some not, run the gamut from blue collar to white, and everything in between. Think firefighters, chefs, nurses, day traders, painting-and-roofing contractors, moving-company honchos. The lawyers and doctors buy, but rarely stay. There is even a retired protestant bishop, who's a Parkie like me.

Cigar smoking is backdrop to the Humidor's main but mostly unspoken purpose. It's a "Cheers Bar" place.

Regulars who still have hair, let it down. The conversation mix at the bar is mostly personal: estrangements, divorces, children, retirement, news of the weird, Bucs doings, the Rays playoff chances.

Politics talk is muted, especially since the divisive election of 2016. The very racially diverse regulars steer away from conversational flashpoints. Respect is a Humidor shared value.

Humidor camaraderie is medicine for the soul, and sometimes even more.

"I can no longer afford my anti-depressant medication," says Mikey, the Humidor's unofficial social chairman. "I treat my depression by being here."

A Mikey specialty is baseball outings—beer, food, cigars at George Steinbrenner Field.

Conversation is easy. "You never meet a stranger here," says deputy sheriff Robert.

"We're family," says Grandpa Ron.

The Humidor family has tended to me since my Parkinson's diagnosis in 2014. Dropped pills. Man bag left atop my SUV. Misplaced lighters. They police my forgetfulness and inattention.

That's you Mike and Mikey, Brian, Shel, Dennis, Harry, Pepsi Ron, Chuck, Coach, Dave and Dave, Todd, Steve, "Bish," Reggie, Curtis, and so many more.

I wrote this to the guys on the occasion of my departure from Tampa to Macon in November.

"You have been there for me, ups and downs, lost gear, withdrawn, exuberant.

"Please select a special cigar as a small measure of my gratitude for your compassion and fellowship over years together at the Humidor Clubhouse for boys (mostly) of all ages.

"Present this card at the cash register as payment in full.

"With deepest regard,

"Gil"

I love Tampa Humidor and all it represents

For me, the Humidor is a place to write, read, quip. It's a second home filled with delightful friends.

As my PD has ebbed and flowed, my mates have recovered things I dropped (most famously my wedding ring into a stuffed chair), helped me recover rolling pills and see to it that I leave nothing behind.

As we prepare to leave for our new home in Macon, GA, I know there will never be another Tampa Humidor in my future.

I love it for what it stands for and the many friends who make it so very special.

Adios, guys.

Early Diagnosis Matters

By Carolyn Allen Zeiger, Ph.D.,
retired Licensed Psychologist and spouse of someone with
Parkinson's Disease

In Parkinson's Disease, early diagnosis does matter—for some obvious reasons, and also for reasons that are rarely discussed.

The question I always hear people with Parkinson's (PWPs)—and their spouses—ask about someone else with PD is not, "How long have you had PD?" but "When were you diagnosed?" Given that there is no definitive medical test to confirm the diagnosis, the delay between symptom onset and diagnosis is generally a few years. The thinking used to be that an early diagnosis didn't matter. After all, at this time it can't be cured, it's going to progress, and perhaps it is best to delay the use of dopamine replacement medications since they only provide symptom relief. In addition, even some physicians still harbor the mistaken belief that these medications tend to lose their effectiveness over time. Generally unstated, is also the thought that early in the progression of the disease it doesn't have a big negative impact on the patient, or his life in general. He's doing well enough to get by. But is he or she? And what about the spouse or partner?

Fortunately, more doctors are focusing on early diagnosis. But not for a reason that I find compelling: the impact of PD on our most intimate relationships—spouse, partner, lover. So many times

I have heard, and experienced myself, the painful impact of undi-agnosed PD on our closest relationships. Sometimes the impact is so great as to mean the ending of even long-term marriages when unidentified symptoms become burdensome or sources of ongoing conflict.

The precise source of the problems varies depending on the varying symptom patterns. Here are just a few stories:

Facial masking. A wife wept as she told me, "He never smiled at me anymore. I kept asking, are you angry with me? Don't you love me anymore?" He didn't know what I was talking about. Finally he did get angry. "Just leave me alone! Nothing is wrong." She began to pull back; he responded in kind. A long time, close and open relationship became distant and closed off.

Fading Voice. When the PWP can't be heard, he feels ignored, or is convinced that his partner has a hearing problem because he is not aware that his voice has become soft. His speech might be slurred and hard to understand as well. His partner becomes impatient, and perhaps a little embarrassed, so she begins to speak for him; the PWP pulls back, goes silent and a destructive pattern has been established.

Apathy. Partner: "Get off that couch and DO something! All you do is sit around."

PWP: "But I don't feel like doing anything."

Partner: "If you would just get moving, you would."

But no amount of either nagging or kind encouragement makes a difference because the apathy has a neurological basis. The spouse starts doing things by himself because "Nothing I do gets her moving, and I don't want to stay home all the time." Both are lonely.

REM Sleep Behavior Disorder. During the night, a man is awakened by his wife screaming and swearing at him. He's completely shocked and furious. "I didn't do anything to deserve that!" When he wakes her up, she doesn't have any idea what he is talking about. Another PWP punched his sleeping wife—convinced he was actually "saving her from a gorilla". Of course the gorilla was in a dream that he was unknowingly acting out.

Of course, symptoms interact and exacerbate each other.

Foot dragging combined with fragmentation of sleep at night and daytime fatigue can lead to frequent tripping and falls, injuries that put a burden on them both, and lead to injuries and/or health problems for the partner as well as the PWP.

In all these scenarios, the accumulation of seemingly minor symptoms can lead to a major disruption in the relationship. The partner with PD feels constantly scrutinized, unfairly criticized, and nagged. The care partner feels ignored, disbelieved, and abandoned. Over time, both partners may feel mistreated or simply neglected. The distance and constant tension of conflict, even low-level conflict, erodes the intimacy in the relationship.

One of the areas where couples experience the most pain is in the most intimate relationship: sex. Many aspects of PD can interfere with a couple's sex life. They include fatigue, apathy, loss of erectile function, reduced libido, and anxiety. All are neurologically based symptoms that can appear to be psychological (and might be that as well!), or stem from something going wrong in the relationship. Some of the physical symptoms such as awkward movements, loss of bladder control or drooling can be embarrassing or repellant to either one of them. The result is that either partner may pull away or give up. Talking about it is important, but isn't sufficient to solve the problems when the cause remains a mystery to them both.

In talking to both PWPs and their partners, I very rarely hear about a doctor inquiring about a couple's sex life—before or after diagnosis. Sometimes younger clinicians assume that an older couple doesn't have a sex life any longer. Or the couple might think they are just "too old" now, so they don't even think to tell the doctor. For younger couples this can be even more disruptive to the relationship. As a psychologist, I know this is a difficult subject for any patient to broach, whatever their age or stage in life, and so it is seldom addressed.

What can be done?

More doctors understand that PD is more than a movement disorder. Some are taking a whole-person focus and inquiring about your whole life. This may seem odd or inappropriate—sex is not what you came in to talk about—nonetheless, it is invaluable. You can help the clinicians out by telling them everything that is bothering you, whether you consider it physiological or psychological. Because my husband's symptoms were more autonomic than motor, no doctor would consider evaluating him for PD, even when asked. Nevertheless, because a nurse asked us to tell her everything we were concerned about, the interview revealed the pattern of autonomic as well as movement related disorders that characterize PD.

And after you receive a diagnosis, continue to report all your concerns—both partners' concerns. Because the PWP is often not aware of his symptoms, the perspective of those closest to him is essential for both diagnosis and selection of the best possible treatment of symptoms. Also what bothers the partner may not bother the PWP and vice versa. Both of you count.

Read books that focus on all aspects of living with PD, such as Brain and Behavior by Joseph H. Friedman, MD, and 100 Questions and Answers about Parkinson Disease by Abraham Lieberman, MD. I highly recommend getting the Phinney Foundation guide Every Victory Counts. Read and contribute to blogs that focus on PD.

Talk about your relationships in support groups. I have found other members are so relieved to have someone bring up difficult topics, to know they are not alone, and are grateful to other members who share ideas and approaches that are helpful.

Have your support group leaders bring in experts to talk about the impact of PD on relationships—including sex. When I have given such talks, some members begin to talk openly while others sit quietly listening. Participants share their pain, fears, confusion, guilt, and then sigh with relief as they come to understand what is going wrong and ways to address it. Afterwards, both the quiet and the talkative participants tell me how much it has helped them.

Share this article with neurologists to help them understand more about how PD impacts relationships and the value of early diagnosis. We health professionals truly want to be helpful, and to do so, we need to educate and consult with each other.

Medication may provide "only" symptom-relief, but relief can be essential to restoring and preserving your relationship. Also, treatment is more than medication. It includes exercise. Exercise of various kinds has been shown to not only improve function, but to stimulate neural growth. In our work teaching yoga for Parkinson's, our students reported that it improves mood and self-confidence (And we could see it!). Just having fun is therapy! Treatment can also include support groups and psychotherapy, enjoyable activities—anything that improves your quality of life.

A combination of treatments tailored to the individual PWP, taking into account the person's life situation and key relationships, provides a better quality of life for everyone, both individually and as a couple. Improvement in one aspect of your life starts a positive feedback loop, and each person's life becomes more satisfying!

Carolyn Allen Zeiger, Ph.D. has over 45 years' experience in the fields of clinical, organizational and health psychology. With Kate Kelsall's husband, Tom, she founded a Parkinson's care partners' support group in Denver, and assisted her husband Paul in teaching yoga to others with Parkinson's Disease and their partners. Carolyn is a retired State of Colorado Licensed Psychologist, and former adjunct faculty member at University of Denver, University of Colorado and University of Arizona. She also provided short term counseling for the caregivers of those with Parkinson's Disease.

Your Health-Care Network

Physician Resources

- Primary care physician/Internist/Gerontologist

- Movement Disorder Specialist (MDS) Neurologist

- Neurologist

- Neuropsychologist

- Gastroenterologist

- Urologist

- Sleep specialist/doctor

- Endocrinologist

- Psychologist/Clinical Psychologist

- Neurosurgeon

Health Professional Resources

- Physical therapist

- Occupational therapist

- Speech pathologist

- Fitness/Personal trainer

- Nutritionist

- Masseuse

- Palliative care counselor

- Social worker

Personal Support Resources

- Family

- Friends

- Community organizations

- Spiritual resources

- Support group(s)

- Exercise classes

- Computer brain games

- Financial adviser

- Legal adviser

[Expanded from PD SELF's Health-Care Team and personal experience.]

Palliative care for Parkinson's disease: suggestions from a council of patient and care partners

By Kirk Hall, Malenna Sumrall, Gil Thelen, Benzi N. Kluger and on behalf of the 2015 Parkinson's Disease Foundation sponsored "Palliative Care and Parkinson Disease" Patient Advisory Council

Abstract

In 2015, the Parkinson's Disease Foundation sponsored the first international meeting on Palliative Care and Parkinson's disease and the Patient Centered Outcomes Research Institute funded the first comparative effectiveness trial of palliative care for Parkinson's disease. A council of Parkinson's disease patients and care partners was engaged to assist with both projects. This council wrote the following manuscript as an opinion piece addressed to the clinical and research community on how palliative care could be applied to people living with Parkinson's disease and their families. The council endorses palliative care as an approach to the care of Parkinson's disease patients and their families that seeks to reduce suffering through spiritual, psychosocial, and medical support. This approach should start at the time of diagnosis, as this is a very challenging time for patients and care partners; includes better emotional support, educational resources, and closer follow-up than is currently standard; and continue through end-of-life care and bereavement.

Thomas Graboys, M.D., was a beloved Boston cardiologist who struggled for years with Parkinson's disease (PD)-related dementia. He died with it in 2015. His book, Life in the Balance: A Physician's Memoir of Life, Love, and Loss with Parkinson's Disease and Dementia, bared his innermost thoughts about what having Parkinson's and dementia feels and looks like. As a physician, he believed in sensitive and effective patient care. His life story and clinical philosophy strongly influenced our thinking on PD palliative care.

When the doctor's verdict is rendered "PD" is a day we patients will never forget. For some, there is a momentary sense of relief that the accumulating symptoms have a cause and name. For others, the reaction is terror, shock, and confusion. We ask, "What does this diagnosis mean for me?" Few receive information beyond the diagnosis on what PD is, what we can do about it, and what our future holds. Commonly, we leave the doctor's office on our own with a levodopa prescription and instructions to return in 3 months.

How would Graboys have broken the news of a Parkinson's diagnosis if he had been a neurologist and not a cardiologist?

He would take the time to explain what PD is, encouragement about available therapies, and information about the importance of exercise and diet. Graboys would tell us that patients who do well with PD do not let it own them. "You don't have to do this alone," he would say. Graboys would also explain at a meeting 1 month later how there was an organization we could join with educational seminars, programs for care partners, and recommendations for physical and other therapists. He would work closely with the organization to see that care provision was modified as needed for each of us. Graboys would write out any medications he recommended and explain what they were for. He would discuss exercise, diet, and other lifestyle changes that would help enhance our life. He would call it the "plan."

It was this contract between Graboys and the patient that, if adhered to, would reduce stress and increase the chances of a positive outcome. And because the plan was personal, it was more likely to be honored. Just leaving the office with that plan in hand inspired hope because implicit in that plan was the message that there were things the patient could do to take control of his/her illness and enhance his/her chances of living a fairly normal life.

The Graboys allegory contains many of the early stage recommendations of our own prescription for PD Palliative Care and is based on the approach Graboys took with his own patients. While such an approach may not fit every physician or patient, we hope it provides some useful examples of patient-centered care for PD.

The Patient Prescription for PD Palliative Care was created by PD advocates Kirk Hall and Gil Thelen based on their personal experiences and personal interaction with other patients and care partners. It outlines recommendations for changes or incremental actions to improve patient quality of life. It is not intended to be an indictment of the current system or the dedicated practitioners who operate within it.

We envision a new, improved approach to Palliative Care based on a "three-legged stool" including the patient's primary care physician and neurologist (leg 1), a PD palliative care team (leg 2), and a PD support entity (leg 3). The "three legs" are meant to provide support for patients, care partners, and families throughout the PD journey.

Early stage: diagnosis to 5 years (honeymoon period)

Given confusion and misperceptions about palliative care, we suggest using the term "supportive care" and discussing this concept as PD Life Enhancement, or something similar. Palliative care should provide a comprehensive, coordinated, and consistent approach for the medical and PD support communities designed to maximize quality of life for patients, care partners, and families starting at diagnosis and to reduce stress for the duration of the disease and bereavement period.

The key points for diagnosis were included in the Graboys allegory. Another important element is sharing informational resources (see Appendix 1 for an example). We recommend scheduling follow-up a month after diagnosis since many patients are "shell-shocked" and unable to absorb much beyond the words PD. This is an opportunity for the doctor to assess how the patient and care partner are doing, ask if they have reviewed information resources, and answer questions.

The potential value of support groups should be discussed. Finally, it is important for the doctor to outline what information to bring for future appointments to make appropriate care decisions.

We recommend an appointment a year after diagnosis to assess the patient's and care partner's "readiness" to be provided with additional informational resources (see Appendix 2). Most people should be ready at that point and some may have already begun this process on their own. If not, we recommend discussing why they are not ready. Some patients take the "what I don't know won't hurt me" approach. It is important to share that in general, patients and care partners who do best in managing PD take "ownership" of it so that they can properly advocate for themselves and make good choices. We recommend participation in self-efficacy or chronic disease management education programs. This is also a good time to revisit the potential benefits of joining a support group. The doctor should have a working relationship with regional and local support groups.

We propose that at some point in the first couple years following diagnosis, the person with Parkinson's (PWP) and care partner should be asked what they know about palliative care. If they have attended a self-efficacy program, they may know a great deal. Make sure that they understand how it works and the benefits of such a program, emphasizing the need to get involved prior to late stage symptoms in order to avoid unnecessary stress and confusion.

Middle stage: 5 years to advent of symptoms that substantially affect daily living

The middle stage is a crucial time for patients, care partners, and families. It is a time when learning can take place relative to late stage. Plans and decisions can be made to make the later stage easier. Wrestling with these issues, including faith, can create acceptance and peace of mind, making the last stage of the journey far less stressful.

Tasks should include:

A personal plan for taking ownership of possible outcomes, including the possibility of financial challenges.
Develop end of life wish list and legal documents including advance directives.
Discuss with doctor what his/her role will be in end stage.
Discuss care partner plan for assistance and self-care.
Begin assessing need for in-home safety and for equipment.
Consider counseling to address faith/spiritual issues or concerns.

Many patients, care partners, and families miss this extremely important opportunity for a variety of reasons. They may not have as much warning as they think before they are in the thick of late stage and end up scurrying around to find resources, fighting among themselves at a time when they need to be focused on caring for each other. They may not want to face the inevitable decline of their loved one and the difficult decisions this entails, so they take the "ostrich" approach by sticking their heads in the sand. PD palliative care clinics may have value in helping families in this stage.

Late stage: advent of significant disability/ hospice to death/bereavement

In our model, the late stage becomes a matter of implementing plans and preferences identified in the middle stage including hospice when appropriate. Legal paperwork will be available to minimize confusion, misunderstandings, or other "bumps in the road." Of course, it is not likely that all developments can be foreseen and planned for, but these should be the exception. If the plan includes contingencies based on the nature of specific health issues as they unfold, there can be "course adjustments" as opposed to confusion and stress related to confrontation of unanticipated issues.

We recommended that the patient's primary neurologist stay engaged with the patient and care partner in late stage. By that time, a significant relationship based on experience and trust has often been created with both the patient and care partner. If not, following the Graboys allegory, it should have been. From our perspective it seems that many neurologists are uncomfortable remaining involved after they can no longer "fix" their patient. Training in palliative care or involvement of palliative medicine specialists could help remedy this issue.

It is extremely important to be mindful of care partner stress/ burnout at this stage, and this is an area where a palliative care team could and should add great value. The team needs to be aware that the care partner can become so overwhelmed that they do not take the time or have the energy to reach out for help. A regular "check-in" should be established that, if missed, would trigger contact by the team. Finally, while bereavement is easy to overlook, we must be mindful of the needs of the care partner and families following the death of the patient.

PD support organization proposal

In order for the three-legged stool concept to work consistently and to facilitate development and implementation of programs as well as sharing of best practices, we recommended development of a unified regional program coordinated by a single national entity. Based on our information and experience, we recommended the approach taken by Association of Independent Regional Parkinson Organizations as a model that allows for autonomy and at the same time keeps the benefits of being part of a group, such as timely sharing of information and learning from fellow members' successes and failures. As a model for a single region, the Muhammad Ali Parkinson's Center in Phoenix is one potential candidate.

Medical community proposal

We proposed a fundamental shift in the mindset and training of doctors starting in medical school to facilitate the changes discussed, including getting to know patients and care partners beyond their medical records and the importance of remaining engaged in late stage to help ensure a "successful transition to death." We would describe this as one in which the care partner, family, and medical team can feel at peace because they did everything possible to honor the patient's wishes about how he/she wanted to die.

This raises an important topic in the minds of the overwhelming majority of PD patients that needs to be resolved. For most of us, it makes no sense to prolong suffering for patients and, in the process, impose huge medical bills on our families by not giving us the choice to die, when no hope of a cure remains. We deserve to have all reasonable choices available to us without risking a stain on our legacies.

Another recommended area of focus for medical schools is the ethical aspects of working with patients who would be better served elsewhere. This is a sensitive subject because it shines a spotlight on doctors who choose to continue treating a patient despite knowing better options exist. We have seen many patients in our support groups receive inappropriate treatments or be incorrectly told there is nothing more to offer by doctors without PD-specific knowledge or skills.

Finally, we add our voice to the many who have called for development of telemedicine and other technologies to increase access to high-quality care in remote/rural areas and for patients with mobility issues.

Conclusions

Needs and gaps include:

"Palliative Care" terminology confusion

Team approach to palliative care

Reduction of diagnosis angst

Planning for end stage beginning in middle stage

Early and better utilization of hospice

Role of neurologist in late stage

Patient control of the manner in which they die

Care partner/bereavement needs

Remote area needs

High-priority areas for future research include:

1. Identify barriers and opportunities in the medical community to implement palliative care.

2. Determine the impact of the implementation of the new approach to PD palliative care on PWP, care partner, and family's quality of life at each stage of the disease.

3. Determine the effectiveness of new and existing remote area care alternatives to deliver palliative care.

4. Learn from other palliative care approaches (e.g., cancer) that might improve PD palliative care.

References

1. Graboys, T. Life in the Balance, (Union Square, 2008).

2. Hall, K. Window of Opportunity: Living with the Reality of Parkinson's and the Threat of Dementia, Chapter 13: Palliative Care and Neurology: Striving for Justice, (North Slope Publishing, 2014).

3. Boersma, I., Miyasaki, J., Kutner, J. & Kluger, B. M. Palliative care and neurology: time for a paradigm shift. Neurology **83**, 561–567 (2014).

Acknowledgments

The authors dedicate this manuscript to the memory of Dr. Thomas Graboys who was generous with his time in developing these ideas when he was alive and who continues to inspire us in our work. The authors would like to thank the other members of the patient advisory council (Fran Berry, Linda Hall, Carol Johnson, Candace Maley, Pat Maley, and Marilyn Villano) for their support and input. This work was supported by the Parkinson's Disease Foundation Conference Grant (Palliative Care in PD) and partially supported through a Patient-Centered Outcomes Research Institute (PCORI) Award (IHS-1408-20134). The statements in this article, including its findings and conclusions, are solely the responsibility of the authors and do not necessarily represent the views of the PCORI, its Board of Governors or Methodology Committee.

Author information

Affiliations

Parkinson's Disease Patient and Advocate, Highlands Ranch, CO, USA - Kirk Hall

Carepartner for Parkinson's Disease Patient and Advocate, Castle Rock, CO, USA - Malenna Sumrall

Parkinson's Disease Patient and Advocate, Tampa, FL, USA - Gil Thelen

Movement Disorders Center, University of Colorado Denver, Aurora, CO, USA - Benzi M. Kluger
Consortia
On behalf of the 2015 Parkinson's Disease Foundation sponsored "Palliative Care and Parkinson's Disease" Patient Advisory Council.

Contributions

K.H., manuscript concept and creation of first draft; M.S., revision of manuscript; G.T., revision of manuscript; B.M.K., clinical and editorial contributions to manuscript.

Competing interests

The authors declare no competing interests.

Corresponding author

Correspondence to Benzi M. Kluger.

Supplementary information

Appendix 1 (which follows)
Appendix 2 (which follows)

[Web links accurate at time of article publication, 22 May 2017.]

Journal Article Appendix 1:
Newly Diagnosed Parkinson's Education & Resources

This resource guide has been assembled by an experienced patient/care partner group and members of the Parkinson's disease (PD) medical/research community who share a common goal, which is to improve quality of life for people with Parkinson's (PWPs), care partners, and their families. A common concern of the newly diagnosed is how to find the information that they want and need. In this brochure are links to resources that we have found helpful to provide basic information regarding Parkinson's, including young onset. In the future, we hope a comprehensive guide will be available that would allow you to access a wide range of additional information. If you are unable for any reason to obtain information you seek, there are services (e.g. local support groups, national organizations) that will enable you to speak directly with someone who can help.

But first, our PWP/care partner members want to share a few things they have learned that we think are important for you to know:

Give yourself some time to "process" your diagnosis. This is a major unanticipated change in your life. It is natural to have some feelings of fear and anxiety, but remember you can take ownership of this process. Yes, your life will be different, but you will be surrounded by many people in support groups, PD organizations, and the medical community who are dedicated to making your life better! Not to mention the support of family and friends (the same people you would support if they were going through something like this). As soon as you are ready:

Your #1 priority is to be sure you are working with a doctor that has appropriate experience, training, and education for your condition. Do not assume that your doctor, no matter how much you may like him or her, meets this description! Not all neurologists, for example, have movement disorder expertise that will enable them to recognize the subtle symptoms of PD and recommend appropriate medications and/or therapies. If your doctor is not a good fit for you, or even if you are not sure and want a second opinion, we will provide information in our resource guide to help you locate a movement disorder neurologist in your area.

Your #2 priority is to understand that exercise has been proven to be an effective way for you to improve your condition and how you feel as well as potentially slowing the progression of the disease. It will help you stay positively engaged and fight off the apathy that some of us experience. Work with your doctor to determine what kinds of exercise would be best for you.

Your #3 priority is to take ownership of your situation by learning about PD and how you can live well with it. This will enable you and your care partner to take an active role in the management of your condition, including providing information about your symptoms (include all symptoms, whether or not you think they are related), any changes you have experienced, things that concern you, medications you are taking, other conditions you may have, and more. If you have concerns, ask questions! If your doctor consistently does not take the time to answer your questions, find a new one! Your obligation is to yourself and your family!

Your #4 priority is to locate and join a PD support group. "Test drive" one or two, if necessary, to find one that is comfortable for you and your care partner. If you have trouble locating a support group, contact your regional support organization for suggestions. Get involved!

If you are in a remote area, your options may be limited. We know people who have teamed with a local neurologist working in conjunction with a movement disorder specialist that you can visit occasionally. Another option is telemedicine, which allows you to receive care using communication technology. Explore these options with your doctor to find an arrangement that works for you.

Stay engaged! The steps above will get you moving in a positive direction. With PD there are good days and bad days. Just know during a bad day that the good days will come back. Own each bad day and don't let it turn into a bad week. You do not have to go through this alone!

There is a need for newly diagnosed patient participation in clinical research! To learn more visit https://foxtrialfinder.michaelj-fox.org/register/ and complete the profile.

Resources

Help locating a movement disorder neurologist and why this is important

- Michael J. Fox Foundation (MJFF): https://www.partnersinparkinsons.org/find-movement-disorder-specialist?cid=aff_00032
- Parkinson Disease Foundation (PDF): http://www.pdf.org/spring12_specialist

Exercise information

- Davis Phinney Foundation (DPF): http://www.davisphinneyfoundation.org/living-pd/10tools/?gclid=Cj0KEQjw75yxBRD78uqEnuG-5vcBEiQAQbaxSNfO0tFlTMxBMKAMkKJ6jp6-tzI7Y4nwRBFoEliVcgcaAkdv8P8HAQ
- Brian Grant Foundation (BGF): http://www.briangrant.org/
- National Parkinson Foundation (NPF): http://www.parkinson.org/understanding-parkinsons/treatment/Exercise/Neuroprotective-Benefits-of-Exercise
- Parkinson Disease Foundation (PDF): http://www.pdf.org/en/parkinson_exercise_impact

Newly diagnosed information

- Parkinson Disease Foundation (PDF): http://www.pdf.org/symptoms

- National Parkinson Foundation (NPF): http://www.parkinson. org/understanding-parkinsons/what-is-parkinsons
- Michael J. Fox Foundation (MJFF): https://www. michaeljfox.org/understanding-parkinsons/index. html?navid=understanding-pd
- American Parkinson Disease Association (APDA): http://www.apdaparkinson.org/parkinsons-disease/ understanding-the-basics/

Young onset information

- APDA: http://www.apdaparkinson.org/ national-young-onset-center/
- NPF: http://www.parkinson.org/understanding-parkinsons/ what-is-parkinsons/young-onset-parkinsons

Help locating a support group (PWP & care partner)

- NPF: http://www.parkinson.org/find-help/ resources-in-your-community
- PDF: http://www.pdf.org/en/support_list
- APDA: http://www.apdaparkinson.org/resources-support/ local-resources/
- PDF: http://www.pdf.org/en/airpo

Help locating a care partner support group

- Parkinson's Health (PH): http://www.parkinsonshealth.com/ Caring-for-Someone-with-PD/Support-Groups.aspx

Talk directly to a person who can help

- NPF: http://www.parkinson.org/find-help/helpline
- PDF: http://www.pdf.org/en/ask_expert
- MJFF: https://www.partnersinparkinsons.org/ parkinsons-advocate-program?cid=aff_00032

[Web links accurate at time of article publication, 22 May 2017.]

Journal Article Appendix 2:
Parkinson's Education & Resources:
1+ years since diagnosis

This resource guide has been assembled by an experienced patient/care partner group and members of the Parkinson's disease (PD) medical/research community who share a common goal, which is to improve quality of life for people with Parkinson's (PWPs), care partners, and their families. We designed it for PWPs and care partners who are not considered "newly diagnosed" (typically one year since diagnosis).

We want to make it easier for you to find the information and resources that will make it possible for you to be informed and advocate for yourselves effectively. The good news is that, thanks to the dedication of Parkinson resource organizations, just about any information you may need is available on their websites. The problem is that, for many of us, the specific information we seek is not always easy to find within those websites.

Others may not be armed with enough information to know what they should be looking for.

This guide will provide links to topics that are important for all "seasoned" PWPs and care partners to understand. That said, we also want to equip you to find information you seek on almost any topic related to PD. Using your favorite internet search engine (like Google at www.google.com), enter Parkinson's and _____ (any topic such as fatigue, driving, care partner issues, depression, anxiety, sleep issues, etc.) in the search box and click "Enter" on your computer keyboard. A list of information resources will appear. Some of the information may not be reliable, so pay attention to the source.

Much of the reliable information will be from PD organizations or medical websites such as Parkinson Disease Foundation (PDF), National Parkinson Foundation (NPF), Michael J. Fox Foundation (MJFF), the Mayo Clinic, National Institutes of Health (NIH), and more. Since developments and new information are ongoing, note the date of articles to see which are most current. Another tip to get the most current information is to type in the current year (i.e. 2015) after your subject title in the search box.

But first, we want to share our recommendations and experiences for living well with PD:

Continue to make exercise a priority.

Learn about palliative care. Check out the palliative care links in the resource list below.

Attend programs provided in your area that explain palliative care and why it is important.

Participate in clinical research trials. When you do this, you accomplish two things. First, you help with the advancement of knowledge that will lead to a cure. Second, you learn things that may help you. Information on specific studies, including availability, location, and timing of research trials can be found at https://foxtrialfinder.michaeljfox.org/.

Learn everything you can about PD. This applies to both PWPs and care partners. By doing this, you will have a better idea of what to expect in terms of symptoms and progression. Also, it will enable both of you to advocate for yourselves, ask informed questions, and become active/proactive in the management of your health.

Prepare for your doctor appointments. Remember that doctors are very busy individuals who want to provide you with the best care possible. Help make the limited time you have together in appointments productive by preparing a list that includes your current prescriptions, supplements, and symptoms; observations/information regarding your condition; and a list of questions regarding your condition, symptoms, treatment, medications, alternative therapies, or new developments you have heard about that may apply to you.

If you are not comfortable with your doctor for any reason, talk to him or her about it. If you are unable to resolve problems that are important to you, find another doctor! Your number-one obligation is to yourself and your care partner.

Set meaningful goals and work to accomplish them. If this has always been your approach, continue it. If it has not, resolve to start. Hold yourself accountable and ask your care partner to do the same.

Stay in touch with your passions. Some of the non-motor problems associated with PD can include depression, anxiety, and apathy. You may be able to reduce these kinds of issues by engaging in activities that have been important to you in the past.

Communicate with each other. It is crucial to keep the lines of communication between you and your care partner open. Tell each other what you are thinking and feeling. Share the things you are worried about and problem-solve together.

Attempt to "live in the moment" as much as possible. Learn from the past and move on. Plan for the future, but do not dwell on the uncertainty that it surely contains.

Balance. Your "PD life" takes place in the context of your overall life. It will be beneficial for both of you to keep the two integrated and balanced as much as possible.

Perspective. Continue to find the joy in your lives. Celebrate the small victories. Do NOT let PD own you!

Take care of yourself (care partners). Ask for help. Solicit assistance as needed from family members and/or friends. Make time for yourself. Stay engaged with your passions. Attend to your personal wellness.

Patience (care partners). PD mood swings and/or cognitive problems can be very hard on relationships. No matter how good your communication, it is likely that your partner will sometimes act or react in ways that are not tactful or appropriate. Try very hard not to take these things personally. At a later time, communicate about what happened if you can.

Resources

Apathy/importance of staying engaged

- http://movementdisorders.ufhealth.org/2013/11/26/apathy-and-parkinsons-disease/

Care partner wellness

- https://www.michaeljfox.org/foundation/news-detail.php?parkinson-disease-information-for-carepartners-and-loved-ones&smcid=ag-a30U00000004i07&s_src=adwords&s_subsrc=adwords_caregiving_blogpost&smcid=ag-a30U00000004i07&gclid=Cj0KEQiA4LCyBRCY0N7Oy-mSgNIBEiQAyg39thb6-0J405edhuIKbtDTD-9bX599AzU0L0n1jFj2jiwaAsLK8P8HAQ
- http://www.pdf.org/en/caregiving_fam_issues?gclid=Cj0KEQiA4LCyBRCY0N7Oy-mSgNIBEiQAyg39ttgyKIq8S-bGBTZxzchsp6Se_32dkxELj7Mqx972qMcaAoJb8P8HAQ
- http://www.pdf.org/en/coping_skills_parkinson_carepartner
- http://journals.lww.com/neurologynow/Fulltext/2015/11030/Anger_Management__Many_neurologic_conditions_can.14.aspx

Deep brain stimulation

- http://www.parkinson.org/understanding-parkinsons/treatment/surgery-treatment-options/Deep-Brain-Stimulation
- http://www.ninds.nih.gov/disorders/deep_brain_stimulation/deep_brain_stimulation.htm
- http://www.pdf.org/en/surgical_treatments?gclid=Cj0KEQiA4LCyBRCY0N7Oy-mSgNIBEiQAyg39tgjM4e6gh53Rgp0sSALEdyZy7T22Tj4eRL_baPidUFsaAnIQ8P8HAQ

Depression/Anxiety

- https://www.michaeljfox.org/understanding-parkinsons/living-with-pd/topic.php?emotions-depression

- http://www.pdf.org/en/combating_depression
- http://www.parkinson.org/understanding-parkinsons/non-motor-symptoms/anxiety/What-are-the-Treatment-Options-for-Anxiety

Driving

- http://www.pdf.org/parkinson_briefing_driving?gclid=Cj0KEQiA4LCyBRCY0N7Oy-mSgNIBEiQAyg39trxo7KzWfjTzg26fvtgXt5OWnDaLAS2NTBjjVVag9asaAlUh8P8HAQ
- http://www.parkinson.org/understanding-parkinsons/living-well/activities-of-daily-living/driving-with-pd

Dyskinesia

- https://www.michaeljfox.org/understanding-parkinsons/living-with-pd/topic.php?dyskinesia&smcid=ag-a30U00000004hVt&gclid=Cj0KEQiA4LCyBRCY0N7Oy-mSgNIBEiQAyg39thoaSYHh-rXNhafs6Rjo10B1966_I7nn3LXESTKIb70aAme28P8HAQ

End of life issues/planning

- http://hospiceandlifecarecenter.org/reso/begin-conversation/?gclid=Cj0KEQiA4LCyBRCY0N7Oy-mSgNIBEiQAyg39tnISsba05cM1DCA5N27C-z7pBC5_hWxQSyxaO9I7PZ4aAkMG8P8HAQ

Fatigue/chronic tiredness

- http://www.parkinson.org/sites/default/files/fatigue-and-parkinsons.pdf

Gastrointestinal issues

- http://www.pdf.org/en/gastrointestinal_problems_pd

Living well with PD

- http://www.davisphinneyfoundation.org/living-pd/webinar/videos/10-commandments/
- http://www.davisphinneyfoundation.org/living-pd/

Medications/Treatments

- http://www.pdf.org/en/meds_treatments
- http://www.mayoclinic.org/diseases-conditions/parkinsons-disease/basics/treatment/con-20028488

Melanoma

- https://www.michaeljfox.org/foundation/news-detail.php?parkinson-disease-linked-to-melanoma

Motor symptoms

- http://www.pdf.org/symptoms_primary
- http://www.parkinson.org/Understanding-Parkinsons/Motor-Symptoms

Non-motor symptoms

- http://www.pdf.org/symptoms_nonmotor_early
- http://www.apdaparkinson.org/parkinsons-disease-non-motor-symptoms/

Pain

- http://www.pdf.org/en/pain_pd

Palliative care/hospice

- http://www.parkinsonsresource.org/carepartner/quality-of-life-palliative-and-hospice-care/
- https://getpalliativecare.org/whatis/disease-types/parkinsons-disease-palliative-care/

Parkinson's dementia

- http://www.alz.org/dementia/parkinsons-disease-symptoms.
asp
- https://www.nia.nih.gov/alzheimers/publication/
lewy-body-dementia/basics-lewy-body-dementia

Parkinson's psychosis/hallucinations

- http://www.parkinson.org/understanding-
parkinsons/non-motor-symptoms/Psychosis/
What-are-the-Treatment-Options-for-Psychosis
- http://www.pdpsychosis.com/?%2Bparkinsons+paranoiaP
D+PsychosisParanoia&gclid=Cj0KEQiA4LCyBRCY0N7Oy-
mSgNIBEiQAyg39tp8Bq7KgBHsW-PNlfSqJYi89a6xqNLKhbm
E7XZ15d1gaAuyC8P8HAQ#uti-block11

REM Behavior Disorder

- http://www.healthline.com/health/sleep/
rem-sleep-disorder#Overview1

Restless leg syndrome

- http://www.apdaparkinson.org/
restless-leg-syndrome-and-parkinsons-disease/

Sleep issues

- https://sleepfoundation.org/sleep-topics/parkinsons-disease-and-sleep
- http://www.apdaparkinson.org/parkinsons-and-the-night/
- http://www.pdf.org/en/sleep_disturbance

Talk directly to a person who can help

- NPF: http://www.parkinson.org/find-help/helpline
- PDF: http://www.pdf.org/en/ask_expert
- MJFF: https://www.partnersinparkinsons.org/parkinsons-advocate-program?cid=aff_00032

[Web links accurate at time of article publication, 22 May 2017.]

REFERENCES

Andrade, Mario de. "Le temps précieux de la maturité" ("The Valuable Time of Maturity"). *Palatable Pictures Blogspot,* translation by Polina Pen, 26 December 2009. Accessed 6 June 2018. Palpable-pictures.blogspot.com/2009/12/valuable-time-of-maturity-mario-de.html.

Davis Phinney Foundation for Parkinson's. *Every Victory Counts,* Fifth Edition, Eighth Printing, 2017.

Graboys, M.D., Thomas with Peter Zheutlin. *Life in the Balance,* Union Square Press, April 2008.

Hall, Kirk. "Newly Diagnosed Parkinson's Education & Resources." *Shakypawsgrampa.com*, 21 October 2015. Accessed 21 May 2018. *www.shakypawsgrampa.com/index.php/new-blog/entry/newly-diagnosed-parkinson-s-education-resources.*

------------, Malenna Sumrall, Gil Thelen and Benzi M. Kluger. "Palliative care for Parkinson's disease: suggestions from a council of patients and care partners." *Nature*, 22 May 2017. Accessed 21 May 2018. www.nature.com/articles/s41531-017-0016-2.

Khullar, Dr. Dhruv. "How Social Isolation Is Killing Us." *The New York Times*, 22 December 2016. Accessed 1 June 2018. www.nytimes.com/2016/12/22/upshot/how-social-isolation-is-killing-us.html.

Lewis, Thomas, Fari Amini and Richard Lamar. *A General Theory of Love*. Vintage, Kindle edition, January 2001.

MedicineNet. "Medical Definition of Placebo effect." *MedicineNet.com*, last editorial review 13 May 2016. Accessed 21 May 2018. www.medicinenet.com/script/main/art. asp?articlekey=31481.

Okun, M.D., Michael S. *Parkinson's Treatment: 10 Secrets to a Happier Life*. CreateSpace/Amazon, March 2013.

Palfreman, Jon. *Brain Storms: The Race to Unlock The Mysteries of Parkinson's Disease*. Scientific American / Farrar, Straus and Giroux, September 2015.

------------. "The Bright Side of Parkinson's." *The New York Times*, 21 February 2015. Accessed 4 June 2017. www.nytimes. com/2015/02/22/opinion/sunday/the-bright-side-of-parkinsons. html.

Parkinson Alliance. "Survey Examines Social Support in Parkinson's Disease from the Patient's Perspective." *ParkinsonAlliance.org*, 2017. Accessed 1 June 2018. www. parkinsonalliance.org/?s=social+support.

Parkinson's Foundation. "Neuroprotective Benefits of Exercise." *Parkinson.org*, 2018. Accessed 14 May 2018. www. parkinson.org/Understanding-Parkinsons/Treatment/Exercise/ Neuroprotective-Benefits-of-Exercise.

------------. *Parkinson's Disease Q&A*, Seventh Edition, 2017.

PD SELF. "Empowering the Newly Diagnosed." *Pdself.org*, 2018. Accessed 14 May 2018. www.pdself.org/empowering-1/.

Riley, David E. "Non-Motor Aspects of Parkinson's Disease" reworded with permission from "A Great Take on Non-Motor Challenges." *ShufflingEditor.com*, 26

March 2016. Accessed 5 June 2017. www.shufflingeditor.
com/2016/03/26/a-great-take-on-pd-non-motor-challenges/.

Thelen, Gil. "Bow Ties Pummel Parkinson's." *ShufflingEditor.com*,
20 September 2017. Accessed 1 May 2018. www.shufflingeditor.
com/2017/09/20/bow-ties-pummel-parkinsons/.

------------. "Filling A Hole in Parkinson's Care." *The Tampa
Tribune*, 24 January 2016.

------------. "The Tampa Humidor Trumps My Parkinson's."
ShufflingEditor.com, 12 October 2017. Accessed 1 May 2018.
www.shufflingeditor.com/2017/10/12/
the-tampa-humidor-trumps-my-parkinsons/.

University of Florida Center for Movement Disorders and
Neurorestoration. "Michael S. Okun, M.D." *UFHealth.org*, 2018.
Accessed 24 April 2018. www.movementdisorders.ufhealth.org/
team/faculty-fellows/michael-s-okun-md/.

Wadman, Meredith. "The Rogue Protein Behind Parkinson's
Disease May Also Protect Your Gut." Science Magazine, 27
June 2017. Accessed 22 July 2018. http://www.sciencemag.org/
news/2017/06/rogue-protein-behind-parkinson-s-disease-may-
also-protect-your-gut.

Zeigler, Dr. Carolyn Allen. "Early Diagnosis Matters."
ZeiglerWebsource, recent edit 20 February 2018. Accessed 30
April 2018. www.74.82.38.19/zeigerwebsource/pdearly5.html/.
Reprinted version supplied by author.

ACKNOWLEDGMENTS AND AFFIRMATIONS

Struby Thelen—my wife, care partner and co-author—who artfully and graciously learned to accept the irrationalities of the Parkinson's Life.

My daughter Debbie and Bill Champion, early believers in my work who jump-started MOPD with generous support.

My sons Todd, Matthew and Jonathan Thelen, who are always there for Dad.

Hyde Park (Tampa) United Methodist ministers Jim Harnish and Justin LaRosa, who were my spiritual coaches in squaring up with the Beast in my brain.

Mindy Bursten, the uncanny clinical social worker who guided me to a fuller realization of what Parkinson's meant for my thinking life.

Agency 3075, the USF advertising class and its brilliant instructor, Coby O'Brien, who gave birth to the Me-Over-PD (MOPD) concept.

Dr. Michael Okun, who demonstrates what patient-centric, team-based healthcare, should look like. His associate Adolfo Ramirez-Zamora delivers it for me at the University of Florida Center for Movement Disorders and Neurorestoration.

Dr. Lucy Guerra, my invaluable Tampa internist who led the health-care team that guided me through the PD "Lightning Strike" in 2016.

Dr. Matt Lazinski, the voluble USF Physical Therapist who teamed with Guerra to remedy "Lightning Strike" damage.

Jordan Brannon and Tara Schwartz of Tampa Bay Rock Steady Boxing, who selflessly brought the fortifying power of RSB to area Parkies, including me.

Valerie Herraro, Parkinson's widow who drives forward patient agendas in Tampa.

Dr. David Riley, the Cleveland MDS who thinks and writes (on my blog, no less) originally about PD non-motor manifestations.

Dr. Jerri D. Edwards, USF Morsani College of Medicine professor who strengthened our book with painstaking critiques.

Drew Smith, my savvy and invaluable Wing Man on the MOPD project.

The Tampa P-DAGgers, the backbone of MOPD distribution plans. Ray and Deanna Commingore, Dan and Laura Crawford, Phil and Joan Daniel, Jerry and Dottie Iwerks, Lynn Olmstead and Phillip Cuculich, Jon and Pat Pawelkop, Brian and Christine Powlette.

Rich Harwood, the community change master who taught how effective communities are created and sustained.

Allyn DiVito, my high-honors aide-de-camp who has kept the technological wheels on every significant project—journalism and Parkinson's—I have undertaken since 1998.

Davis Phinney and Polly Dawkins, leaders of the Davis Phinney Foundation for Parkinson's, who provided me the honor of being a DPF Ambassador.

Dr. Janelle Applequist, assistant professor at USF's Zimmerman School of Advertising and Mass Communications, who with her students and colleague Dr. Deborah Bowen is bringing MOPD to fruition.

Wayne Garcia, interim director of the Zimmerman School who embraced MOPD and made it a centerpiece of the school's ongoing work.

The Rotary Club of New Tampa, which provided operating funds to begin PD SELF training in Tampa.

Diane Cook who with husband Gary saw to the completion of PD SELF training in Tampa.

Kirk and Linda Hall, my gracious hosts in Denver and staunch supporters when I most needed them.

Dr. Latosha Manning and Margie Moore, Tampa-area PTs who were pioneers in bringing Parkies together for the common good.

The late Thomas Graboys, whose searing memoir of his Parkinson's journey (*Life in the Balance*) prompted me to write *Counterpunch*.

Jon Palfreman, who vividly painted the science of PD (*Brain Storms*) and opened my eyes to its ubiquity of symptoms.

Frank MacDonald, Whitney McMath and Margaret Stothart, virtuoso copy editors.

Larry Hoffheimer, whose Parkinson's Place in Sarasota, FL, gave me a glimpse of what a local PD Center might resemble.

Dr. Robert Hauser (acclaimed USF MDS), who gave unsolicited support to my early blog musing about what was to become the Me-Over-PD database of Tampa health-care providers.

THE AUTHORS

Gil Thelen has been a journalist for more than 55 years, including a prizewinning medical reporter in Washington, a managing editor of *The Charlotte Observer*, editor of two South Carolina newspapers (Myrtle Beach and Columbia) before becoming editor of *The Tampa Tribune* in 1998. He was named to the Florida Newspaper Hall of Fame after his retirement as President and Publisher of the *Tribune* in 2006. He was Clendinen Professor at the University of South Florida's School of Journalism and Mass Communications, 2006-14. Gil was educated at Duke University and Cornell University Medical College. He was diagnosed with Parkinson's in 2014.

He is founder and president of Me-Over-PD, a 501(c)(3) foundation. Follow his Parkinson's journey at www.ShufflingEditor.com.

Cynthia Struby Thelen met her future husband in the newsroom of *The Charlotte Observer*. A graduate of Furman University, she was an award-winning designer or supervising editor at *The Columbia* (SC) *Record*, *The Alexandria* (VA) *Gazette* and *The Charlotte Observer*. While Marketing/Research Manager of *The* (Myrtle Beach, SC) *Sun News*, she edited and designed the book *Hurricane Hugo and The Grand Strand*. Her very first book, in loose-leaf form, was *The Story of My Daddy's Life*, written at "age 9 years and 2 months."

Gil and Struby have two sons, multiple cats, and live in Macon, GA. Gil has two children by a first marriage.

All proceeds from the sale of this book go to the Me-Over-PD Foundation, 4972 Hubner Circle, Sarasota, FL 34241.